PHYSICAL TRAINING

A Fusion of Yoga & Calisthenics Sets to Sweat,
Stretch, and Meditate Every Day

—

BY KUNDALINI RESEARCH INSTITUTE

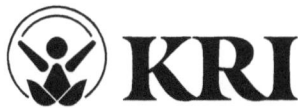

KRI

A KUNDALINI RESEARCH INSTITUTE PUBLICATION

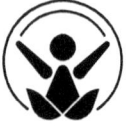

KRI PUBLICATIONS

© 2024 KUNDALINI RESEARCH INSTITUTE

PUBLISHED BY THE KUNDALINI RESEARCH INSTITUTE

TRAINING • PUBLISHING • RESEARCH • RESOURCES

PO BOX 1819 / SANTA CRUZ, NM 87532

WWW.KUNDALINIRESEARCHINSTITUTE.ORG

ISBN: 979-8-9886160-1-6

MANAGING EDITOR: MARIANA LAGE (HARISHABAD KAUR)

CONSULTING EDITOR: AMRIT SINGH KHALSA

COVER AND CREATIVE CONCEPT: FERNANDA MONTE-MÓR

REVIEWER: SIRI NEEL KAUR KHALSA AND LIVDHYAN KAUR

PROOFREADING: CARLOS ANDREI SIQUARA

LAYOUT: CAROLINE GISCHEWSKI

ILLUSTRATIONS: JANIS SOUZA

EDITORIAL ASSISTANT: ANTONIO LARA SILVA

The diet, exercise, and lifestyle suggestions in this book come from ancient yogic traditions. Nothing in this book should be construed as medical advice. Always check with your personal physician or licensed care practitioner before making any significant modifications to your diet or lifestyle to ensure that the lifestyle changes are appropriate for your personal health condition and consistent with any medication you may be taking. Neither the author nor the publisher shall be liable or responsible for any loss, injury, or damage allegedly arising from any information or suggestion in this book. The benefits attributed to the practice of Kundalini Yoga and meditation stem from centuries-old yogic tradition. Individual results will vary.

This publication has received the KRI Seal of Approval. This Seal is given only to products that have been reviewed for accuracy and integrity of the sections containing the 3HO lifestyle and Kundalini Yoga as taught by Yogi Bhajan®. For more information about Kundalini Yoga as taught by Yogi Bhajan® please see **www.kundaliniresearchinstitute.org.**

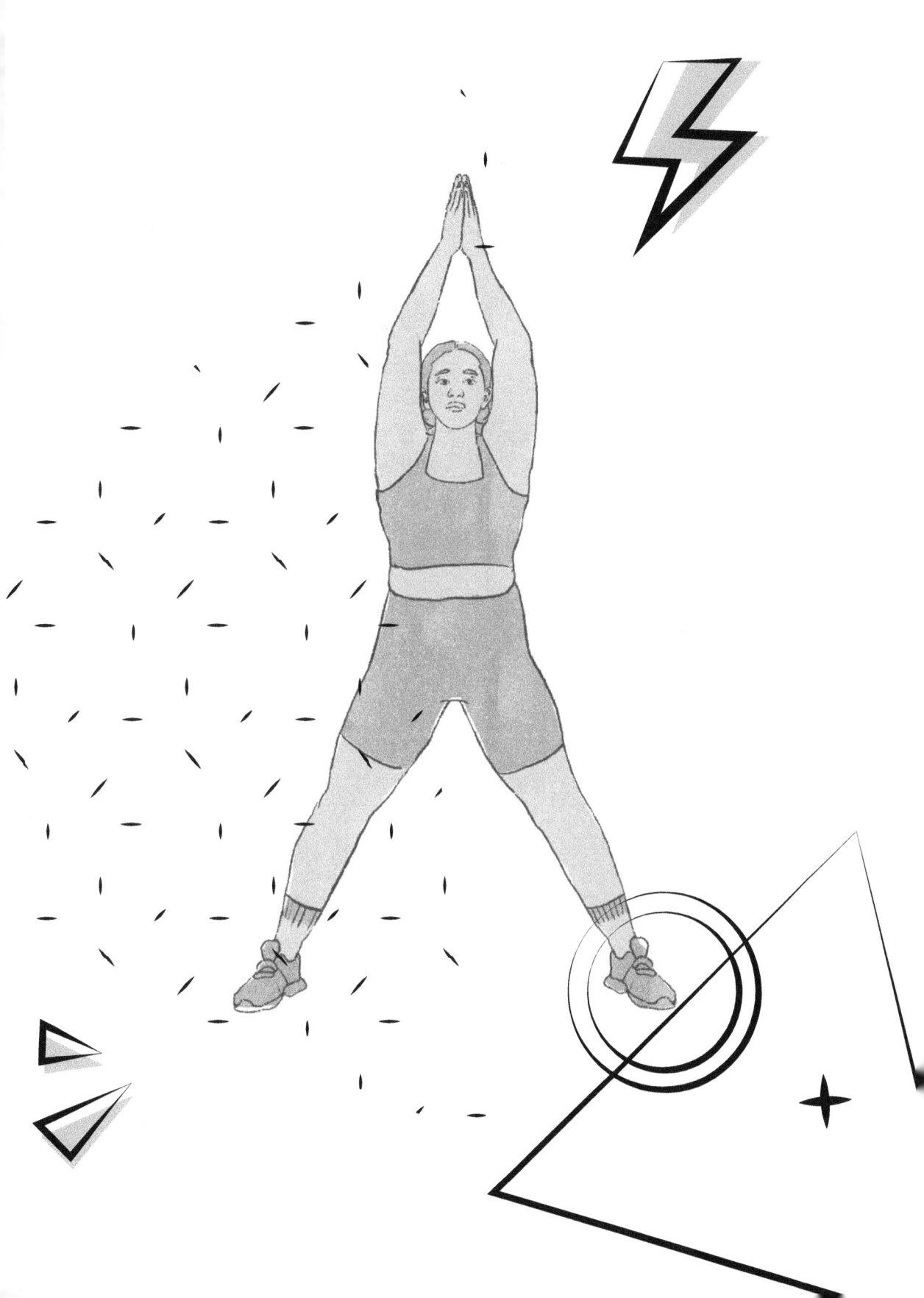

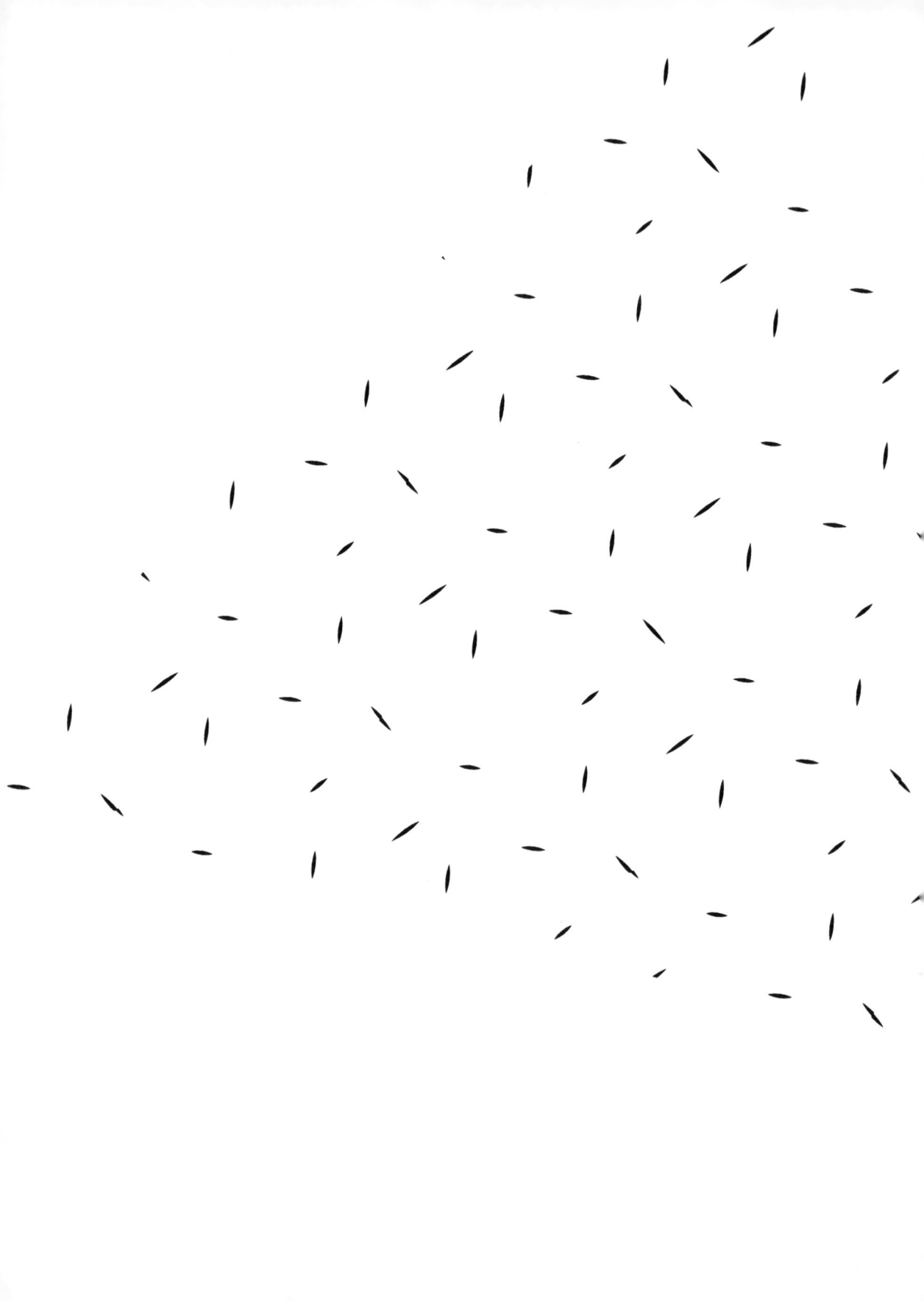

FOREWORD

—

Many Western yoga practitioners have a view of yoga as an exercise practice. It is something that they practice by going to a gym or maybe a dedicated yoga studio. They work out, strengthening and stretching their body, and leave feeling great afterwards.

But the ancient origins of yoga on the Indian subcontinent were much more wholistic. Yoga was typically taught in ashrams to students who were completely immersed in living as yogis 24/7. The end result was always spiritual – the merger of the finite self with the Infinite Self. And that goal was supported by very specific ways of living. Yogis had learned from their own self-experimentation and the long, rich healing traditions (such as Ayurveda) in India: guidelines for every aspect of life (how and what to eat, how to sleep, how to wake up, how to bathe, etc.) that would maximize the practitioner's health, vital energy, and spiritual connection.

Kundalini Yoga as taught by Yogi Bhajan® has a bit of a reputation as a spiritual form of yoga, at least compared with some of the popular Western manifestations of yoga practices. A typical Kundalini Yoga class always includes at least some chanting (at a minimum to tune in at the beginning of class) and some meditating.

Like the original forms of yogic practice, Kundalini Yoga as taught by Yogi Bhajan® involves a lot more than just exercises and meditations taught in a 90-minute class! Yogi Bhajan shared a huge amount of yogic wisdom about other aspects of life that he called "Humanology." This includes all kinds of lifestyle practices that can maximize our physical, mental and emotional strengths and our ability to remain spiritually connected, even under stress or pressure.

The Physical Training exercise sequences in this manual bring us back almost full circle to the western emphasis on yoga being a form of physical fitness. It is, and it is important to keep our bodies strong and healthy! As part of a holistic yogic practice where physical health, mental health, and spiritual connection are all important and mutually supportive, KRI is very excited to bring you this book of physical fitness exercises inspired by ancient yogic practices. We hope that you enjoy using them not to the exclusion of all the other important aspects of yourself, but as an important complement to your life as a balanced yogi.

These exercise sequences are not your typical Kundalini Yoga kriyas. They are exercise sequences, and hence do not need a tune-in before you begin. They represent another unique facet of the vast body of yogic teachings that Yogi Bhajan shared. Practice and share them in health and blessings.

In Service,

Amrit Khalsa, CEO of KRI

TABLE OF CONTENTS

—

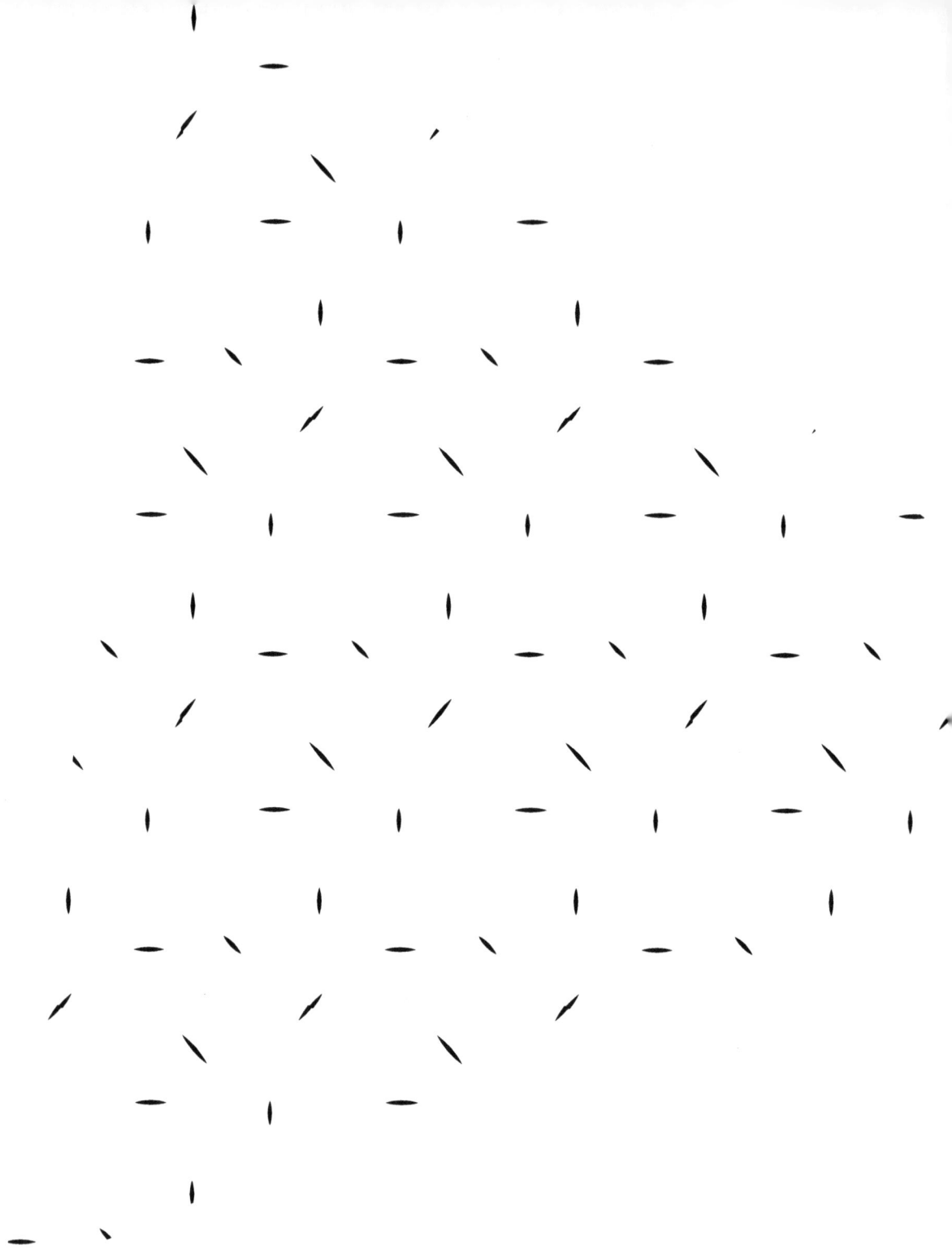

A FUSION OF STRENGTH, RESILIENCE AND WELLBEING

—

Welcome to a transformative journey that combines yoga's ancient wisdom, the energizing power of calisthenics, and the functionality of dynamic movements. These exercise sets are a symphony of intense yet compelling workouts that go beyond ordinary physical exertion and serve as steps towards resilience, strength, and wellbeing, in which breath and movement join to replenish the praana[1] that nourishes your inner being. Engaging in these life-changing exercises can help you to develop not just your physical body but also your spiritual pathways, leading to a life of mindful living, vibrant health, and unmatched fulfillment.

Within this book, you will find a unique collection of workouts from a yogic perspective called Physical Training. These exercise classes were originally taught by Yogi Bhajan during the summers of 1993 and 1994 at what was then known as Ladies' Camp. On weekdays, after morning group sadhana[2] and before breakfast, participants wearing workout clothes and sneakers would engage in these exercise sets outside on a lawn.

Physical Training consists of sets of rigorous, energetic, challenging physical exercises, but they are not *only* physical exercises. They might be called "yogasthenics," a fusion of calisthenics, yoga, and functional movements. Moreover, they combine exercise with yoga practices, so we can sweat, stretch, dance, and meditate every day.

Although the sets may seem simple, they are extremely dynamic and work all of the chakras, the nervous system, the glandular system, and the internal organs. Physical Training is a system for maintaining the person on all levels—physical, mental, and spiritual—to bring out the best in us. Yogic teachings exhort us to keep all levels of the human system clean, so we can

---

1   In yogic teachings, praana is considered the first unit of energy. It refers to the vital life force or energy that permeates the universe and sustains all living beings. It is the fundamental energy that animates our bodies and minds. Prana flows through the body via subtle energy channels called "nadis" and is typically associated with breathing.

2   Sadhana means spiritual discipline. It refers to the early morning meditative practice.

achieve excellence and prevent our bodies from deteriorating as we age. The lifestyle of a Kundalini Yogi involves a daily dose of sweating, meditating and relating to our soul to prevent diverse sicknesses and diseases of the body, mind, and spirit. This book fulfills this intent on all those levels.

While exercise is commonly thought of as "burning calories," the goal of Physical Training is instead to *generate* energy to meet the demands of the day. We burn energy, or consume prana, doing our everyday tasks, so every day prana has to be replaced or refilled to maintain a balance, lest we become depleted and eventually ill. Ancient seekers of this balance developed yoga to restock prana, specifically the practice of pranayam, and to purify the body by cleansing through movement and sweating. Yoga, a union between spirit and body, storage and consumption, creates mentally, physically, and spiritually fit people who can achieve a high quality of life. Elevating ourselves every day is a decision we make for ourselves, something we need to do to keep our pranic balance and avoid being overwhelmed by life, which will allow us to succeed and help others.

Yogi Bhajan reminds us that it is not about how we feel now; it's about how we will feel in 50 years. If we maintain our systems as years are added to our lives, we can continue to feel healthy and strong. To maximize the amount of prana captured, the Physical Training classes were taught under particular conditions: in the early morning and outdoors under the rising sun. Though practitioners may choose to replicate these conditions, you can also choose to practice the way that best fits your routine.

Another purpose of Physical Training is to develop personal discipline because life's challenges demand a very steady presence. With these exercises, you can build mental stamina so you can handle the pressure of life. You can also build physical stamina so you can do what needs to be done. You can build spiritual stamina so you can handle the polarities of life and face the world fearlessly. Doing your best honestly, even when an exercise is hard, develops this discipline. Doing your Physical Training consistently, even when you are short on time or do not feel like it, develops a habit that will help you come through in life.

The practice of Physical Training not only increases physical stamina but also nurtures mental and spiritual fortitude. Each set, each exercise, and each moment of disciplined effort is a step towards a better version of yourself. As you embark on this Physical Training journey, remember that the power to change, to grow, and to achieve resides within you. The practices in this book will help maintain a strong, healthy, and resilient body, mind, and spirit. The consistent practice will replenish your prana, invigorate your essence, and help you face life's challenges with unwavering strength.

We hope you take this invitation, embrace the fusion of calisthenics and yoga, and make a commitment to yourself. Every day, let your body sweat, stretch, dance, and meditate. Elevate yourself, because you deserve a life filled with vitality, excellence, and service to others.

Unique Aspects of Physical Training

As these classes were originally taught right after morning sadhana, participants had already done at least 30 minutes of physical yoga, and, as these sets can be energetic and rigorous, we recommend that you always warm up before beginning. For your convenience, we added three options of warm-ups to this collection of Physical Training sets.

Based on video recordings, we know that someone often led the group in warm-ups and a series of exercises before Yogi Bhajan arrived and began to teach. This is the case of the class from July 21, 1994. If you watch the video on the Library of Teachings for this class, at the very beginning, you will see someone leading exercises as Yogi Bhajan arrives. As these extra exercises were frequently not recorded, we could not include them. What you see in this book is only what Yogi Bhajan taught, which we can accurately describe from the existing videos.

The last set in this book from July 29, 1994, on page 222, was the final Physical Training class Yogi Bhajan taught, and he suggested that students practice this series at home daily. If you have done this whole book and want a practice to carry forward, this set is a good choice.

MEDITATING IN THE SUN

"Sit in the Sun" is one exercise that is unique to Physical Training. In this exercise, energies from the sun are absorbed into the body system, specifically energizing the Third Eye Point and the minor chakras in the palms. This practice is healing and can refresh and rebuild all the cells of the body. Specific pointers Yogi Bhajan gave for this type of meditation include:

» Take off any glasses.
» Move any hair away from the forehead so the sun can strike it.
» Tilt the forehead and the palms so the sun strikes them.
» If you are unable to do this exercise in the sun, simply get into the posture and imagine the rays of the sun warming your forehead, eyes, and palms.

MORNING DEW

As mentioned, these yogasthenic sets were taught in the morning after sadhana and before breakfast, around 6:45 a.m. Working out early in the morning provides for contact with the dew that gathers on the grass overnight. Many ancient cultures and spiritual practices involve bathing in or collecting dew on the body. For instance, the ancient Essenes used to roll naked in the morning dew, a practice to recharge and rejuvenate the body. They believed that morning dew contained parts of the Cosmic Father and Mother Earth, the union of the two seemingly opposed principles from which liquid gold could flow as it grasped the elusive moment of the first ray of light.[3]

The Renaissance Swiss physician Paracelsus believed the dew on vegetation possessed the healing energy of the plants as well as the various planets in the sky. Other traditions and cultures[4] believe that the dew on grass may act as a conductor to help transmit the healing energies of our magnetic earth and the universe. Notably, Bach's floral remedies draw inspiration from this concept, centering on the idea that dew captures the essence of diverse flowers. Dr. Edward Bach, the credited English physician behind the renowned

---

3 Meurois-Givaudan, Anne, and Meurois-Givaudan, Daniel. *The Hidden Face of Jesus from Essene Memory*. Amrita Editions, 1991.

4 For more information about working with dew, please see Plau Brown, *Weatherwatch: The magical properties of dew*, The Guardian, 14 Mar 2011, in https://www.theguardian.com/news/2011/mar/14/weatherwatch-dew-alchemy-magic and Rebecca Ryan, *Walk With Me: Dew Walking Hydrotherapy*, in https://steemit.com/esteemapp/@rebeccaryan/walk-with-me-dew-walking-hydrotherapy-e6af3d449b534

Bach flower remedies, proposed the notion that the dew settled on a flower possesses the therapeutic energies inherent to that specific bloom. He further postulated that the consumption of dewdrops could potentially restore balance to key emotional energy patterns. Body contact with dew is thought to

- » Strengthen the immune system and build resilience;
- » Ensure reflexive strengthening of the abdominal organs;
- » Help combat headaches;
- » Ground energies;
- » Strengthen the muscles of the feet, tendons and ligaments;
- » Straighten the arch of the foot and thus prevent fallen arches and flat feet;
- » Serve as a venous and calf muscle pump;
- » Massage the foot reflex zones;
- » Help relieve stress;
- » Help combat foot perspiration and prevent athlete's foot.

BREATH AND PAUSES BETWEEN EXERCISES

Breath is usually not specified in the Physical Training exercises. Find out how to breathe with the movements for yourself, unless otherwise stated in the instructions.

Unlike Kundalini Yoga kriyas, in which a moment or a few minutes of rest are included to process and integrate the experience of an exercise, most of the Physical Training sets were taught with no pauses or rests between the exercises. For this reason, at the beginning of each set, you may find the statement, "There are no pauses between exercises unless indicated." If there was a rest break after the end of the exercise when it was originally taught, the directive "relax" will appear after the instructions for that specific exercise. If there were no breaks between exercises at all in the original class, you will find the statement, "There are no pauses between exercises," at the beginning of the set.

MILITARY-STYLE INSTRUCTION

When the Physical Training sets were originally taught, many military elements were included in the experience. Students stood at attention, formed straight lines, frequently arranged by height, made sharp turns, and adhered to verbal commands quickly and in unison. Responding immediately to commands develops self-control, trains the person to take charge of themselves and to move quickly in response to a threat, and encourages the mind to penetrate situations rapidly. From a yogic perspective, another purpose is to experience one's control over the muscles, leading to eventual control of the mind and spirit as well.

Making movements collectively and in unison develops group identity and the ability to act cooperatively. This learning to merge with others in action can help build community spirit and experiences of belonging, which can be a bridge to group consciousness or awareness of the collective nature of consciousness. However, we also know that group identity and acting in concert have a shadow side.

Marching in place or in formation was often included in Physical Training classes. This is used militarily to entrain participants, get them to immediately respond to commands without question, and coordinate personal actions with the group. Although marching is a military practice, there is compelling evidence that it balances the right and left hemispheres of the brain and increases the connective tissue between them. This is one reason why a baby crawls before walking.

Militaristic elements were not included in this book, as we understand they were a very specific feature for the students practicing yogasthenics in those days. If you're using this manual to teach a class, you can choose to use these tools—arranging by height, executing sharp turns, standing at attention, responding quickly and in unison to verbal commands—at your discretion as you sense the specific needs of your students.

WRESTLING

One exercise frequently included in sets is Partner Wrestling and even wrestling yourself, in one case! This may be a way to work out the whole body after doing exercises that target one particular area or system, circulating the energy more widely. It may also help balance polarities because disparate energies are exchanged with a partner while wrestling. Wrestling exercises also give you the opportunity to assess your own strength, to hold your own, to know who you are, and to stand up for yourself – not out of reaction, but because you know who you are and can hold your own. They are an opportunity to be assertive but not act out of anger as in many martial arts traditions.

Like other military elements, these wrestling exercises were another way of teaching students to be able to respond to anything in the moment, like a combination of saint and soldier. While it may sound contradictory, Kundalini Yoga as Taught by Yogi Bhajan values both sides of this polarity – the conscious, mindful action in the world represented by the soldier and the merger into the Infinite consciousness represented by the yogi. The soldier-saint ideal displays royal courage, nobility and radiance.

▲ **These wrestling exercises may not be appropriate in every situation.** Please use judgment about your location and capacity and err on the side of safety before practicing or teaching these. To remind you of that, we added this little icon ▲ close to the wrestling exercises so you remember to use caution. If you happen to be practicing by yourself, you can feel free to skip the wrestling exercises or try to wrestle with yourself.

BHANGRA DANCING

Bhangra is a traditional style of folk dancing from the Punjab region of India that originated as a celebration of the harvest and is characterized by vigorous kicks and thrusting arm and shoulder movements. Bhangra can be a joyful, fun way to workout, and the traditional gestures are thought to have many health benefits, including stimulating lymphatic movement, clearing the lungs, strengthening the circulatory system, lowering blood pressure, burning calories, toning all the major muscle groups, building strong bones, increasing circulation to the breast area, and preventing hardening of the diaphragm.

Many of the Bhangra movements involve the shoulders and rib cage, and these vigorous, repetitive motions can open blockages in these areas, increasing breath capacity, metabolism, and youthful vigor. When the rib cage is blocked, only about one-third of the breath capacity is used, and shallow breathing takes in less prana, opening the physical form to disease and the effects of aging. Yogically, the chest cavity is also said to be where the electromagnetic field directly connects to the physical body. Given that, clearing and expanding the chest cavity contributes to a strong electromagnetic field for strong defenses.

Bhangra dancing can help coordinate and integrate both hemispheres of the brain through bilateral movement, just like marching. It can also help coordinate the mind and body. This concentration and coordination of the mind and body improve general brain function, cognitive ability, and emotional expression. All these contribute to neuroplasticity, the brain's ability to form new neural connections to change and adapt.

In many of the original Physical Training sets, specific arm and hand movements were directed to work specific parts and systems of the body, and dancing was always done to high-energy Bhangra music. If you'd like to have some moves down before integrating them into these Physical Training sets, you can find a lot of great videos on YouTube that can teach you the basics (and beyond) of bhangra.

PUNJABI DRUMS

Punjabi Drums is the name of a recording that was commonly used in Physical Training classes to keep an upbeat, regular rhythm for exercises. This traditional style of drumming is used in the Punjab region of India to express joy and celebrate, as well as in spiritual contexts. On SikhNet's Gurbani Media Center, you can find a similar recording by searching for "Nagara Drum." You can also look on Spotify and YouTube for upbeat bhangra drum music. On Spotify there are plenty of options of playlists with Punjabi drums.

HYPNOTIZE

A few meditations and exercises in Physical Training ask you to hypnotize yourself. Yogically, we are all thought to be in a trance that is creating our own reality, or maya. However, the question is: Is the reality we are creating (or enthralled by) useful, given to us by others, and focused on the outside world? Or is the reality we are creating tuned in to our own selves and to the energy of the divine?

Self-hypnosis practice is designed to teach us how to recognize our trances. We have nested layers of trances; we have the trance of being here in this room; we have the trance of our identity, of our families, of our countries; and many other layers. The way to learn to stay out of those trances that don't serve us is to begin to focus on our own internal energy through the practice of yoga. Through self-hypnosis, we learn what it's like to be free from identification with our ego and learned patterns, even if only briefly. We then have the power to choose trances that are more creative and pleasurable, trances of nobility and respect, and avoid trances of suffering and pain. In all circumstances, we have the capacity to choose to be in bigger trances and expand ourselves or to contract and condense ourselves. The practice of self-hypnosis through yoga helps us consciously choose what reality we create.

Yogi Bhajan said that meditation is nothing but self-hypnosis, and hypnosis is nothing but self-meditation. The unconscious mind can be the worst negative trance, and the answer to this is to self-hypnotize (or meditate) to neutralize it. When we are no longer controlled by the unconscious mind, we can choose how we want to react to each and every moment under the guidance of the neutral mind, heart, and soul. This is called conscious living.

Before You Begin

TUNING IN

If you're already familiar with Kundalini Yoga, you know that before every practice we begin by tuning in with the Adi Mantra, ONG NAMO GUROO DAYV NAMO, the mantra that connects us with our higher self, the source of all guidance. As these yogasthenic sets are seen as more physical training and physical attunement of the body, not kriyas per se, we understand that tuning in is not necessary for these sets of practices. If you feel you want to tune in before practicing, use your own judgment and discretion to decide what is right for you. If you do choose to tune in, we advise you to also close the session by chanting the three long SAT NAAMs or singing the Long Time Sunshine song at the end.

PACING AND TAKING CARE OF YOURSELF

These sets of Physical Training exercises often involve rhythmic movement between two or more postures. Begin slowly, keeping a steady rhythm. Then increase the pace gradually, being careful not to strain. Usually, the more you practice an exercise, the faster you can go. Just be sure that the muscles and joints become warm and flexible before attempting rapid movements. In addition, some of the Physical Training exercises can have a very high impact, such as jumping from one posture to another. Always use your own judgment about what is right for your body and what might lead to injury if attempted. It is important to be aware of your body and responsible for its well-being.

CONCLUDING AN EXERCISE

Unless it says otherwise, an exercise can be concluded by inhaling and holding
the breath for a short time, then exhaling and relaxing the posture. While the
breath is being held, apply the Root Lock, contracting the muscles around the
anal sphincter, the sex organs, and the Navel Point while drawing back the navel
towards the spine. This consolidates the effects of any exercise and circulates the
energy to your higher centers. Hold the breath just beyond a level of comfort.
If you experience any discomfort, immediately release the lock and exhale.

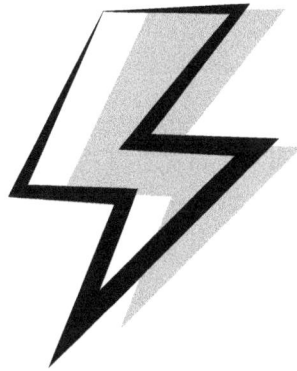
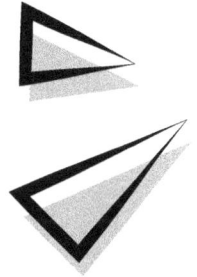

WARM-UP!

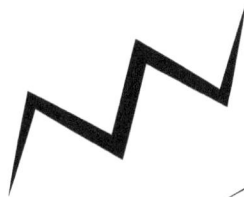
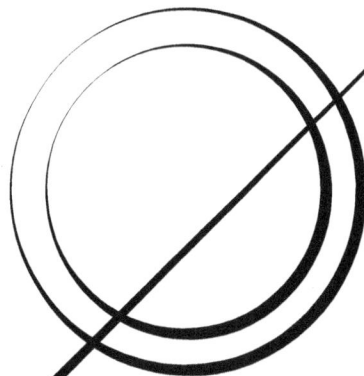
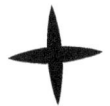

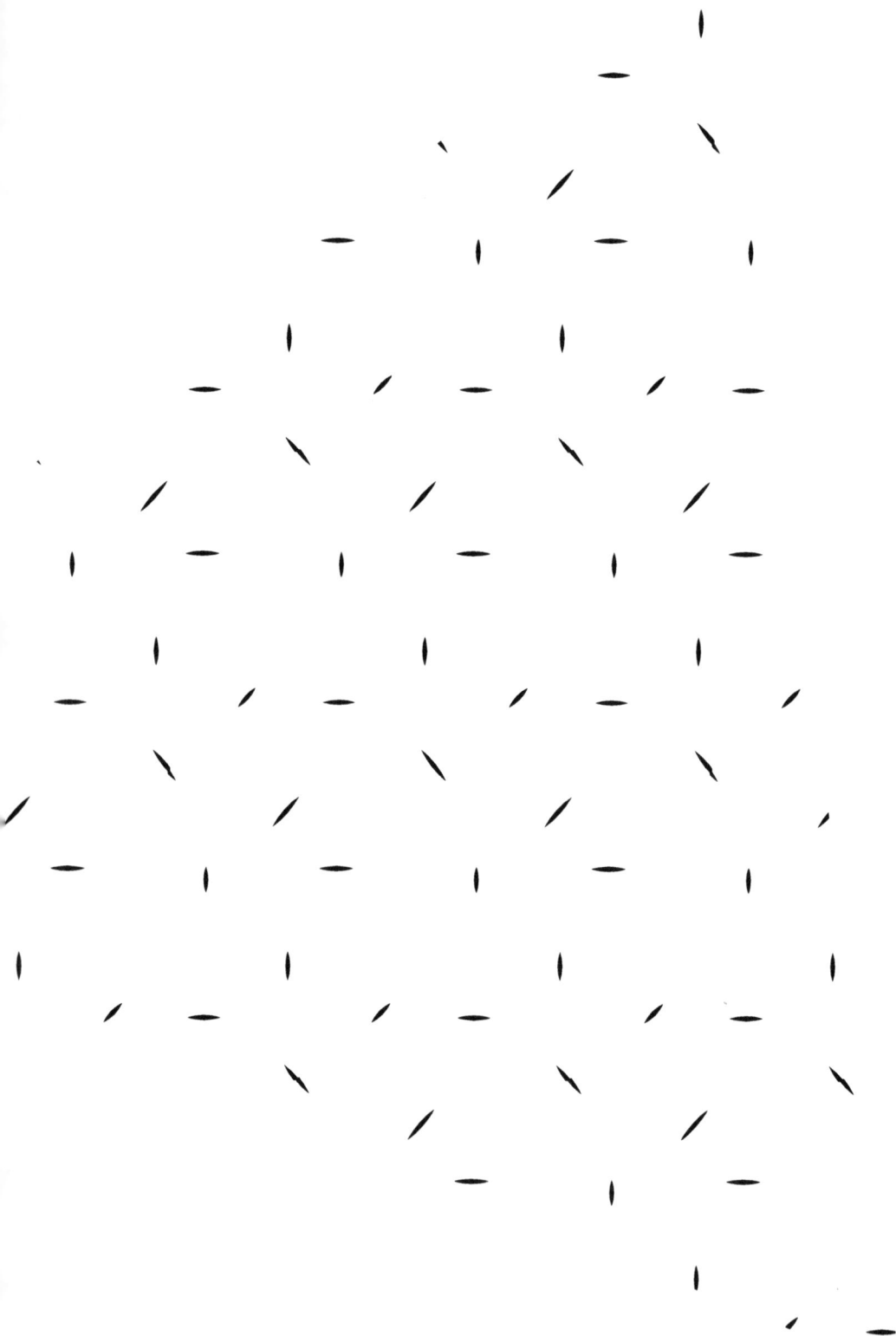

0.1. BREATH OF FIRE WARM-UP

Originally published in The Aquarian Teacher Level 2 — Lifecycles and Lifestyles

1) Sit in Easy Pose with a straight spine and a light Neck Lock. Place your hands in Gyan Mudra on the knees. Begin Breath of Fire and continue for **3 minutes**.

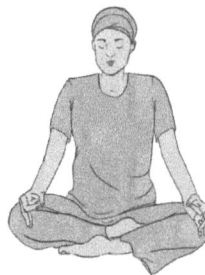

2) Remain in Easy Pose. Extend both arms straight out to the sides, with the palms facing up. Begin Breath of Fire and continue for **3 minutes**.

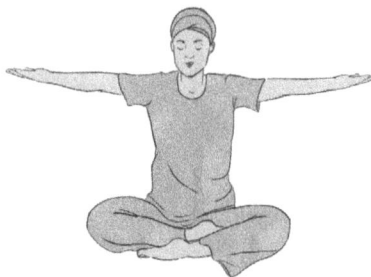

3) Remain in Easy Pose. Bring the palms together in Prayer Pose at the Heart Center. Begin Breath of Fire and continue for **3 minutes**. TO END: Inhale deeply and exhale. Repeat **2 more times**. Relax.

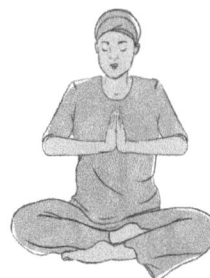

0.2. SPINAL FLEX WARM-UP

Originally published in The Aquarian Teacher Level 2 — Lifecycles and Lifestyles

1) **Yoga March.** Stand up with the feet hip width apart. Inhale and raise both arms straight up, simultaneously raising one leg and bringing the knee up as high as possible. Exhale and bring the arms and leg down. Continue alternating legs for **3 minutes**.

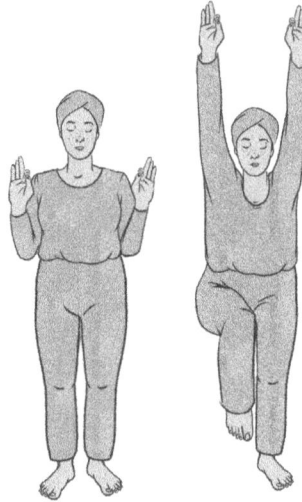

2) **Camel Ride.** Sit in Easy Pose with a straight spine and a light Neck Lock. Grasp the shins or the ankles with the hands. Tilt the pelvis forward on the inhale, lifting the chest up, and backward on the exhale. Only the pelvis and lower spine move. The rib cage, shoulders, and head are still and remain over the hips. The motion is fluid. Continue for **3 minutes** with a powerful breath.

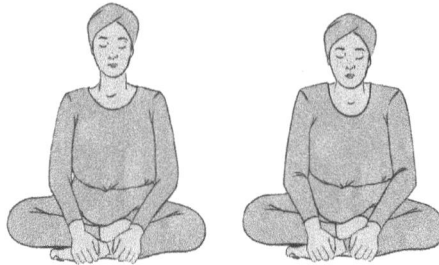

3) **Torso Twist.** Remain in Easy Pose. Grasp the shoulders with the fingers in front and the thumbs in back, and lift the elbows out to the sides and up to shoulder height. Twist the whole torso to the left on the inhale and to the right on the exhale. Keep the upper arms out to the sides and parallel to the ground. The head moves last. The motion is fluid. Continue for **3 minutes**.

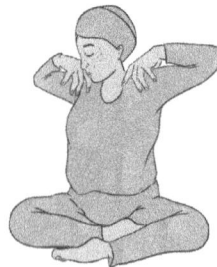

4) **Shoulder Shrugs.** Remain in Easy Pose. Rest the hands on the knees or thighs. Raise both shoulders up towards the ears on the inhale, and drop the shoulders down on the exhale. Move rapidly for **3 minutes**.

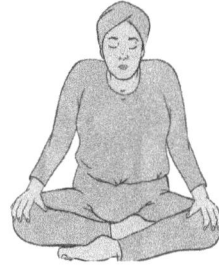

5) **Ego Eradicator.** Remain in Easy Pose. Roll the shoulders down and open the shoulder blades wide. Raise the arms up and straight to 60 degrees. Curl the fingers onto the mounds at the base of the fingers and pull the knuckles back, stretching the palms wide. Draw the thumbs away from the fingers and point them straight up. Keep the neck and shoulder muscles relaxed, and maintain the arms at a 60-degree angle. Close the eyes and focus on the Third Eye Point, while concentrating above the head. Continue for **3 minutes** with Breath of Fire.
TO END: Inhale, suspend the breath, keep the arms straight, and touch the tips of the thumbs together over the head. Open and stretch the fingers wide. Exhale and apply Root Lock. Inhale, exhale, release the Root Lock and slowly lower the arms. Relax.

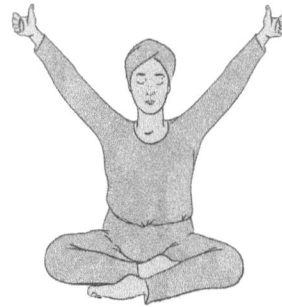

0.3. SURYA NAMASKARA – SUN SALUTATION

1) **Standing Straight.** Stand straight, feet together, toes and heels touching, weight evenly distributed between both feet. Find your balance. The arms are by your sides, fingers loosely together.

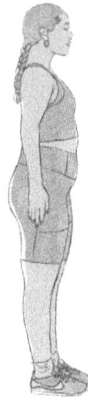

2) **Stretching Up.** Inhale as you bring your arms up overhead, palms touching. Elongate the spine, lift the chest, and relax your shoulders. Be sure not to compress the vertebrae of the neck and lower back. Gaze at the thumbs.

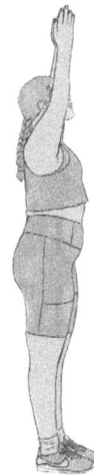

3) **Front Bend.** Exhale and bend your torso forward. As you hinge forward from the hips, keep your spine straight, elongating it as if reaching forward with the top of the head. When the spine can no longer be held straight, relax the head as close to the knees as possible. Ideally, the chin will be brought to the shins. Keep knees straight and place hands on the ground on either side of the feet, with fingertips and tips of the toes in line with each other. Gaze at the tip of the nose.

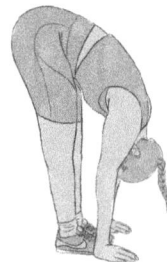

4) **Half Front Bend.** Inhale as you raise the head up, straighten the spine, keeping the hands or fingertips on the ground. Gaze at the Third Eye Point.

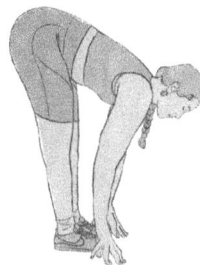

5) **Push-up.** Exhale and bend the knees, stepping or jumping back so the legs are straight out behind, balancing on the bottoms of the bent toes. Elbows are bent, hugging the rib cage, palms are flat on the ground under the shoulders, fingers are spread wide apart. The body is in a straight line from forehead to ankles. Keep equally balanced between hands and feet.

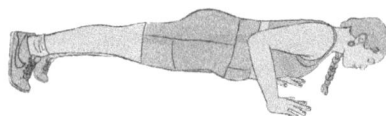

6) **Cobra Pose.** From this position, inhale as you straighten the elbows and arch the back. Stretch through the upper back so that there is no pressure on the lower spine. Lead with the chest, point the forehead up, and gaze at the tip of the nose. Fingers are spread wide apart.

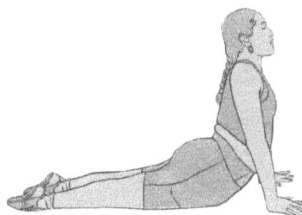

7) **Triangle Pose.** Exhale as you lift the hips up so the body is balanced in an inverted v-shape. Feet and palms are flat on the ground, and elbows and knees straight. Fingers are spread wide apart. Gaze toward the navel and hold this position for **5 breaths**.

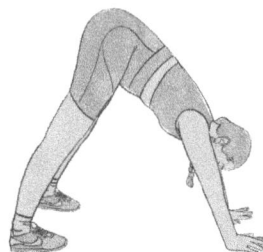

8) Inhale and jump or step back into position #4.

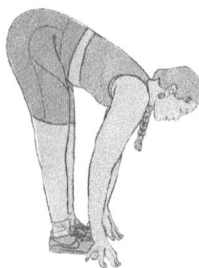

9) **Front Bend.** Exhale and bend forward into position #3.

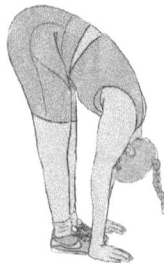

10) **Stretching Up.** Inhale and come all the way up into position #2.

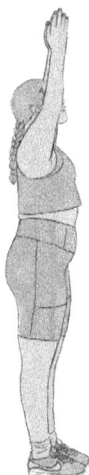

11) **Standing Up.** Exhale and return to the starting position.

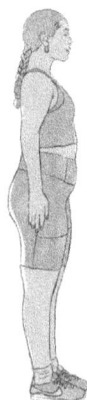

COMMENTS: When Yogi Bhajan was studying with his teacher, the Sun Salutation was used as a warm-up before starting a Kundalini Yoga Kriya. It is an excellent warm-up or can be practiced as a kriya on its own. It increases cardiac activity and circulation, stretches the spine, massages the inner organs, aids the digestive system, exercises the lungs, and oxygenates the blood. When done correctly, the navel and legs do a lot of the work, not the arms and back. Synchronize your breath with the movements to create an uninterrupted rhythm throughout the sequence of positions. Start by practicing three rounds, and then gradually increase to five or six. When practiced with awareness, this improves one's ability to maximize performance and enjoyment of all yoga postures. It doesn't matter if your knees are straight or not; what matters is that your navel moves your spine rather than your head and back. This changes the way you think about everything, creating channels of devotional energy through awareness of body geometry.

① Balance the Energy Through the Chakras

June 9, 1993

There are no pauses between exercises unless indicated.

1) **Kidney Balance.** Stand straight with the feet hip-width apart and a firm Neck Lock. Stretch the arms straight forward from the shoulders, parallel to the ground. Close the eyes and stretch out from the shoulders for **2 minutes**.

2) **Backward Stretch.** Remain in the posture and stretch the arms up and back, bending back slightly. Visualize drawing the energy from the second chakra up the spine. Continue for **1 ½ minutes**.

3) **Wide Leg Half Squat Hold.** Stand with the feet spread wide apart. Stretch the arms straight out to the sides, parallel to the ground. Keeping the spine straight, bend the knees and squat down halfway. Balance in this position for **2 minutes**.

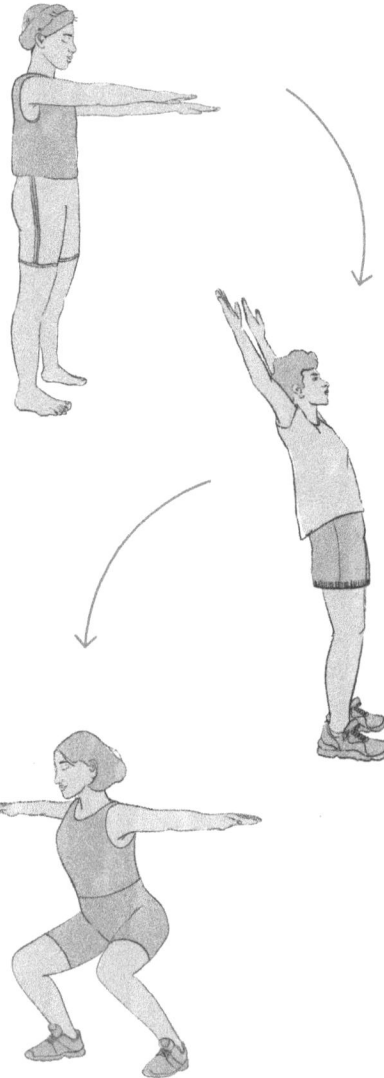

KRI KUNDALINI RESEARCH INSTITUTE

4) **Side Leg and Arm Lifts.** Lie on one side with the head supported in the palm. Lift the leg and arm to 90 degrees and lower them down. Continue rapidly (one lift per second) for **1 minute**. Switch sides and continue for **1 minute**.

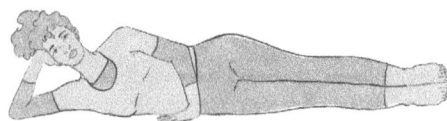

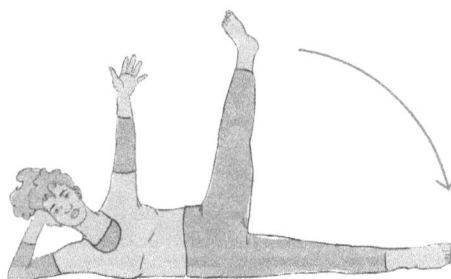

5) **Double Leg Lifts.** Lie down on the back. Raise both legs up to 90 degrees and bring them down. Keep the legs straight and the feet together. Continue at a moderate pace (2 seconds per cycle) for **1 ½ minutes**.

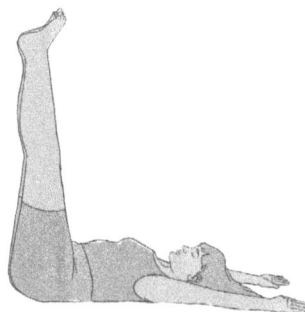

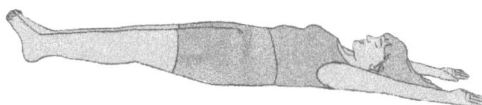

continue on next page »

6) **Push-Ups.** Lie on the stomach with the palms on the ground underneath the shoulders and the toes curled under. With the body held straight, push up on the hands and balls of the feet, then come back down until the chest nearly touches the ground. Continue alternating between the positions for **2 minutes**. Relax.

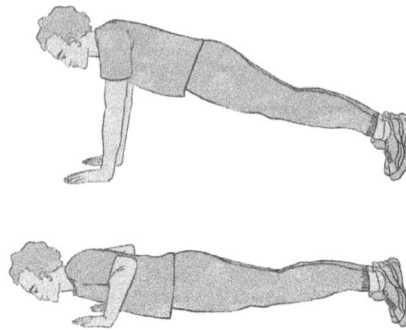

7) **Circle Clap.** Stand with the feet wider than hip-width apart. Clap the hands in front of the upper body. Then circle the arms up, back, and around, coming to the front to clap again, creating the largest circle possible. Chant **HAR** each time you clap and continue (one clap per second) for **1 minute**.

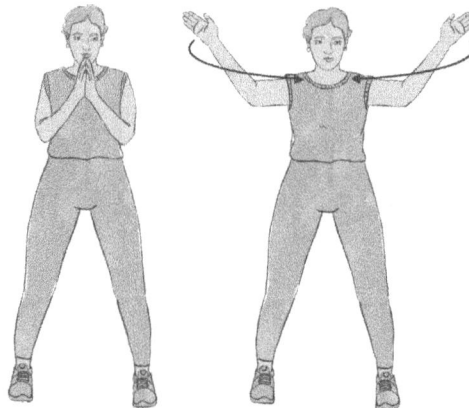

8) **Standing Torso Twist.** Remain in the posture and place the hands on the hips. Twist the torso from side to side and chant **HAR** as you move to the left and the right (one cycle per 2 seconds). Continue for **30 seconds**.

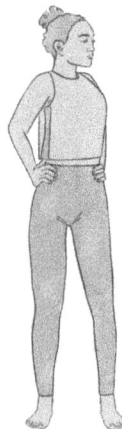

9) **Frog Pose.** Squat down with the heels together off the ground and the fingertips on the ground between the knees in Frog Pose. Chant **HAR** as you straighten the legs and lift the buttocks up, and chant **HAR** as you come back down to the starting position facing forward. Continue alternating between the postures (one cycle per 2 seconds) for **1 ½ minutes**.

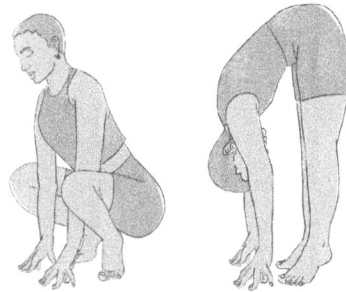

10) **Partner Wrestle.** ▲ Interlock your hands behind the neck of a partner. Try to pull your partner down to the ground without getting pulled down yourself. Continue to wrestle for **3 ½ minutes**. Relax.

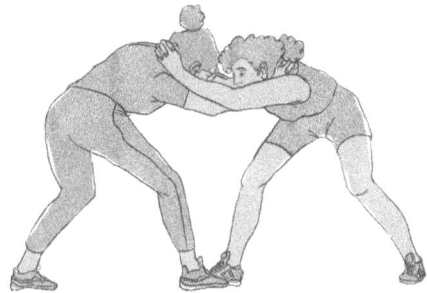

11) **Pelvic Tilt.** Stand with the feet wider than shoulder-width apart and the arms stretched straight out to the sides from the shoulders. Push the pelvis forward and back, allowing the torso to bend forward and back along with the movement while keeping the legs and arms straight. Continue for **1 ½ minutes**.

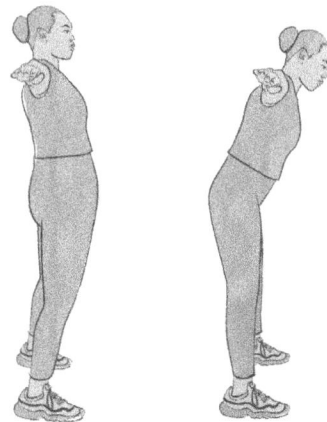

continue on next page »

12) **Eyes Closed Walk.** a) Stand straight with the eyes closed. Find your balance and prepare your mind to guide you by intuition alone for **1 ½ minutes**. b) Walk around your space with the eyes closed, using intuition to avoid others and obstacles, for **1 ½ minutes**. (In the original class, Punjabi Drums were played to keep the rhythm.) *If doing this exercise in a group setting, a few people may protect participants, keeping their eyes open and redirecting others away from obstacles or dangers.*

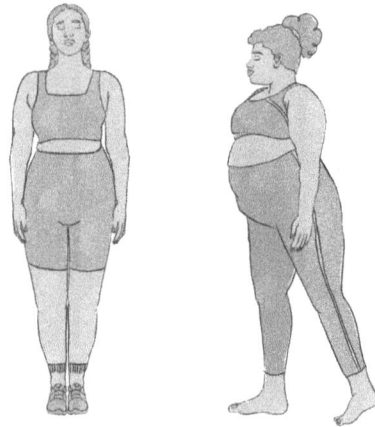

13) **Pelvic Tilt Dance.** Stand straight and bring the hands up above the shoulders. Close the eyes, tilt and move the pelvis in all directions. Shake and dance the pelvis quickly and rhymically for **10 ½ minutes** (you can move the feet and hands as well). (In the original class, Punjabi Drums were played to keep the rhythm.)

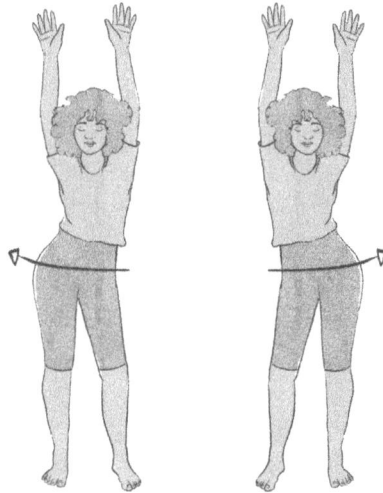

14) **Navel Dance.** Sit in Easy Pose with a light Neck Lock and dance the Navel Point. Keep the rest of the body mostly still as you move and dance the navel around in rhythm for **4 minutes**. (In the original class, Punjabi Drums were played to keep the rhythm.)

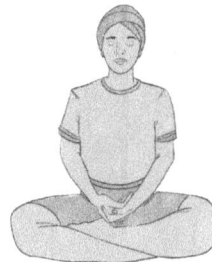

15) **Prayer.** Remain in the posture and pray to God within and without. Continue for **1 minute**.

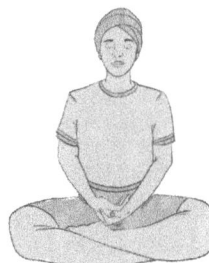

16) **Meditate.** Remain in the posture and meditate. Focus on the relationship between you and the God within you for **3 minutes**. (In the original class, the recording "Rakhe Rakhanhar" by Nirinjan Kaur was played.)
TO END: Laugh loudly for **30 seconds**.

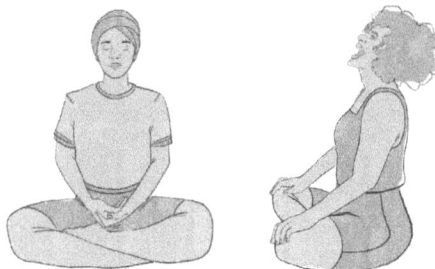

17) **Running.** Run around the space for **2 ½ minutes**.

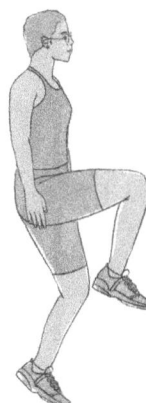

continue on next page »

18) **Sit and Stand.** Stand up straight with the arms straight forward, cross the ankles, and sit down in Easy Pose. Stand up again without using the hands for support. Alternate between standing and sitting (4 seconds per cycle) for **1 minute**. Relax.

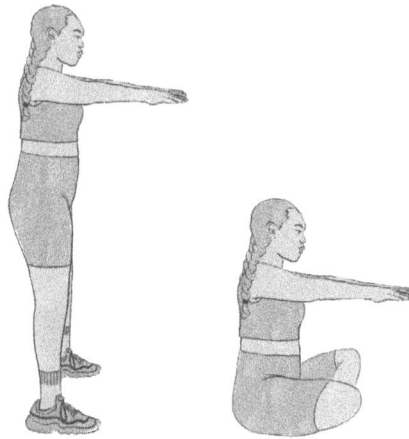

19) **Meditate and Move Kundalini Energy.** Sit in Rock Pose with the knees spread wide, the spine straight, and a light Neck Lock. Place the hands in the crease of the hips and close the eyes. Meditate and move the kundalini energy over the front of the body, from the pelvis up through all of the chakras to the head, over the top of the head, and down the back of the body. Continue for **6 minutes**. TO END: Inhale deeply and exhale two times. Then bend forward, bringing the forehead and hands to the ground. Hold for **30 seconds**.

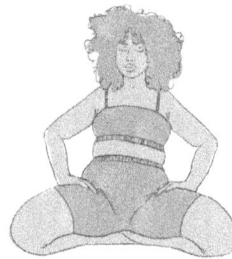

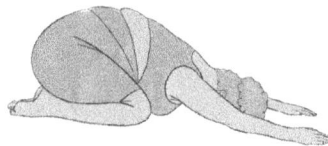

(2) Dynamo Flow and Adrenal Kicker

June 10, 1993

There are no pauses between exercises unless indicated.

1) **Jump Up With Arms.** Stand with the feet hip-width apart. Throw the arms up above the shoulders as you jump up, lifting both knees high. Continue for **30 seconds**.

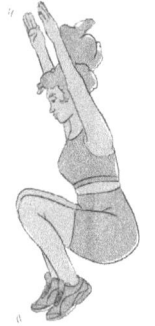

2) **Hip Rotation.** Remain in the posture and place the hands on the hips. Move the hips to the left, to the back, to the right, and to the front. Continue for **1 minute**. Reverse direction and continue for **1 minute**.

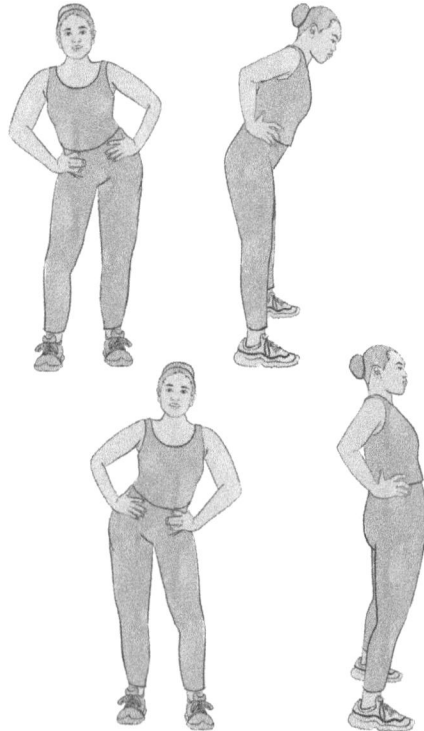

KRI KUNDALINI RESEARCH INSTITUTE

3) **Run In Place.** Remain in the posture and stretch the arms straight forward from the shoulder with the palms facing down. Hold the arms in position and run in place, lifting the knees high, for **1 minute**.

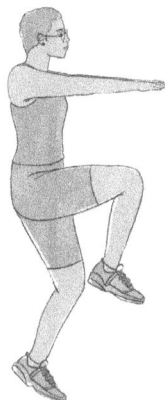

4) **Hop Kicks.** Stand with the feet shoulder-width apart and the hands on the hips. Hop onto one leg while kicking the other leg forward and up parallel to the ground. Continue alternately kicking the legs in rhythm (one kick per second) for **30 seconds**.

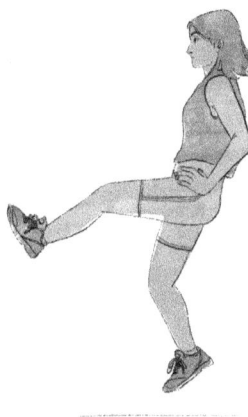

5) **Partner Wrestle.** ▲ Take a partner by the hand and try to bring your partner down to the ground with only one hand. Continue for **1 ½ minutes**.

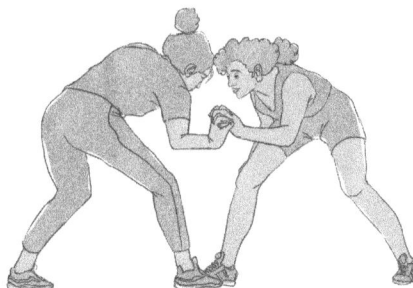

continue on next page »

6) **Frog Jumps.** Squat down with the hands on the ground in front. Jump the feet straight back and place the toes on the ground, then jump the feet back to the squat position. Jump straight up, lifting the knees high, then return to the squat. Continue alternating between the two jumps for **30 seconds**.

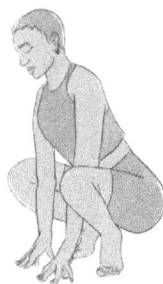

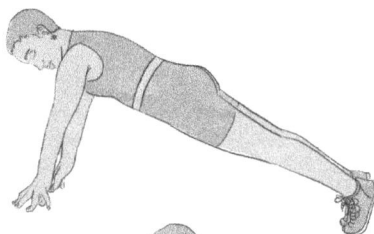

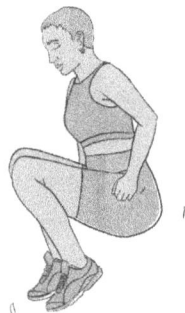

7) **Modified Tree Pose.** Stand straight and bring the sole of one foot to the inner thigh of the opposite leg, or cross the ankle over the opposite thigh. Stretch the arms straight forward from the shoulders and hold the position for **4 minutes**. Switch sides and continue for **30 seconds**. Relax.

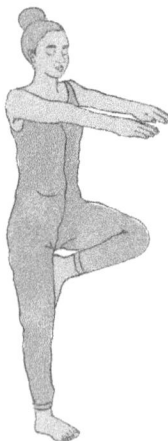

8) **Har Meditation.** Sit in Easy Pose with a straight spine and a light Neck Lock. Chant **HAR** with the tip of the tongue in rhythm at a rapid pace (2 repetitions per second). Pull the navel each time you chant for **2 ½ minutes**. (In the original class, Punjabi Drums were played to keep the rhythm.)

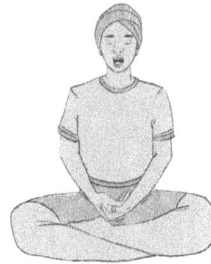

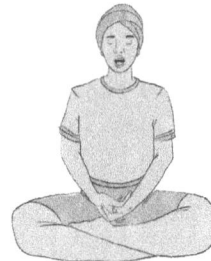

9) **Chant Har Haray Haree.** Chant **HAR HARAY HAREE WHAA-HAY GUROO** in rhythm at a rapid pace (1 repetition per 3 seconds) for **1 minute**. (In the original class, Punjabi Drums were played to keep the rhythm.)

10) **Forward Bend With Crossed Palms.** Come standing up with the legs spread as wide as possible. Stretch the arms forward, palms down, with the right palm on top of the left. Bend forward from the hips until you reach balance. Hold the posture for **2 ½ minutes**. *If you feel dizzy while doing this exercise, sit down immediately.*

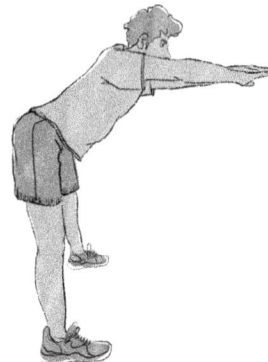

continue on next page »

11) **Backward Stretch.** Keeping the hands and arms as in the previous exercise, stretch up and back. Hold the posture for **1 minute**.

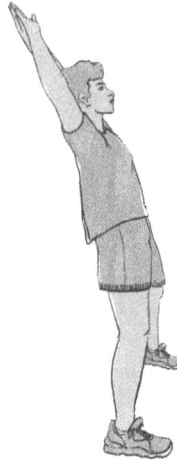

12) **Front Platform Pose.** Come onto all fours and stretch the legs straight back. Support the body on the balls of the feet and the hands. Hold the posture for **1 minute**.

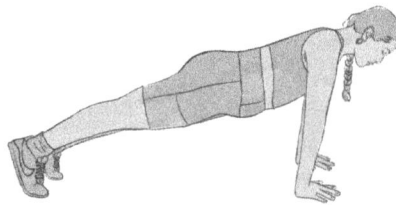

13) **Double Leg Hold.** Lie on the back. Raise both legs to 90 degrees. Hold the posture, keeping the legs straight, for **1 ½ minutes**.

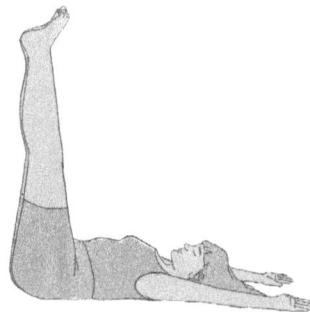

14) **Wide Leg and Arm Hold.** Lie on the back and raise the arms and legs up to 90 degrees, then open them wide. Hold the posture for **1 minute**.

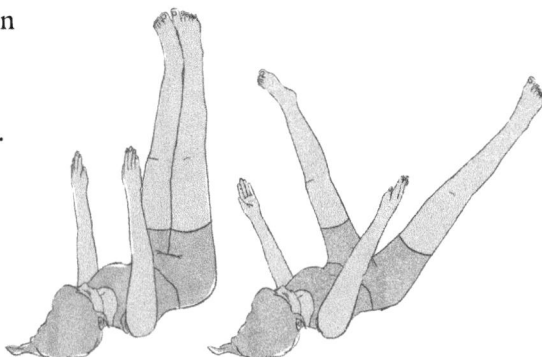

15) **People of Love.** Stand straight with the feet hip-width apart. Raise the arms to 60 degrees. Hold the posture and sing "We Are the People of Love" for **6 minutes**. Relax. *If doing this exercise in a group setting, hold the raised hands of the person on each side.*

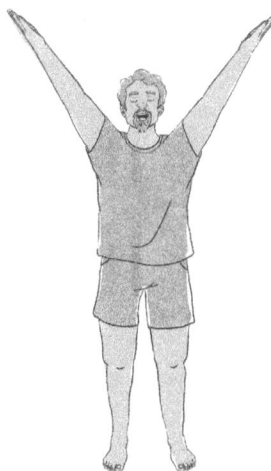

16) **Meditate.** Sit in Easy Pose with a straight spine and a light Neck Lock. Meditate on the strength of your soul for **4 ½ minutes**. Relax.

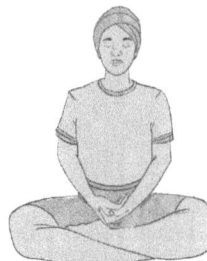

③ Radiant Standing and Seated Series

June 15, 1993

There are no pauses between exercises.

1) Standing Side Bends with Arm Slide. Stand straight with the feet shoulder-width apart. Slowly bend to the left, allowing the left arm to move down the side of the body and the right arm to come up straight. Switch sides and bend to the right. Hold the full stretch on each side for **30 seconds** and continue to alternate for **3 minutes**.

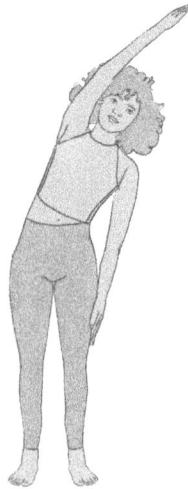

2) Parallel Forward Bend. Stand straight with feet shoulder-width apart. Extend the arms straight up, palms forward. Slowly bend from the hips until the body and arms are parallel to the ground, palms facing down. Stretch forward with the arms and head and backward with the hips. Create a balance. Keep the arms, legs, and spine straight. Continue for **5 ½ minutes**. TO END: From this position, rise up and stretch up and back for **15 seconds**.

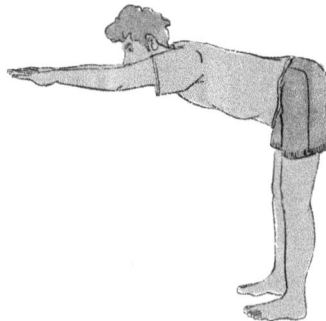

3) **Partner Wrestle.** ▲ Choose a partner and begin to wrestle. Try to take the other person down and pin them to the ground. Continue for **2 minutes**.

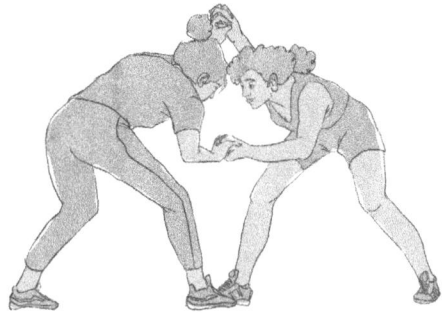

4) **Walk on Hands and Knees.** Come on the hands and knees. Walk around quickly for **1 ½ minutes**.

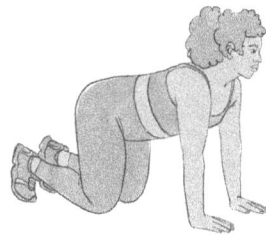

5) **Stand in the Sun.** a) Stand facing the rising sun with the feet shoulder-width apart. Raise the right arm straight up, palm forward. Leave the left arm down with the palm facing forward. Close the eyes and feel the warmth of the sunlight on your forehead, eyelids, and palms of the hands. Hold this position for **3 minutes**. b) Begin to chant **KAL AKAL SIRI AKAL** and alternately raise and lower the arms in rhythm with the palms facing forward. Continue for **2 minutes**. (In the original class, the recording "Kal Akal" by Guru Shabad Singh from the Legacy Collection was played.)

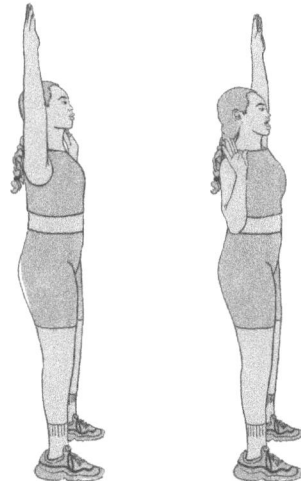

continue on next page »

6) **Sit in the Sun and Dance Series.**
a) Sit in a meditative posture facing the sun. Close the eyes and let the sun shine on the eyelids and forehead. Meditate and move the navel in rhythm for **6 minutes**. b) Without opening the eyes, come standing up. Still facing the sun, dance to the rhythm with the eyes closed for **1 minute**. c) Open the eyes, face a partner, and continue to dance for **5 minutes**. (In the original class, Punjabi Drums were played to keep the rhythm.)

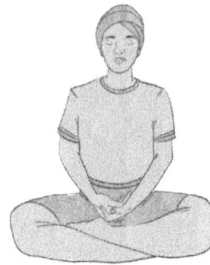

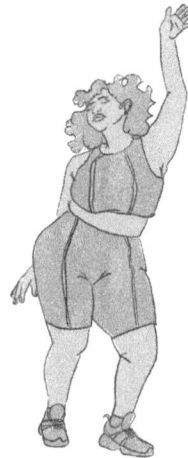

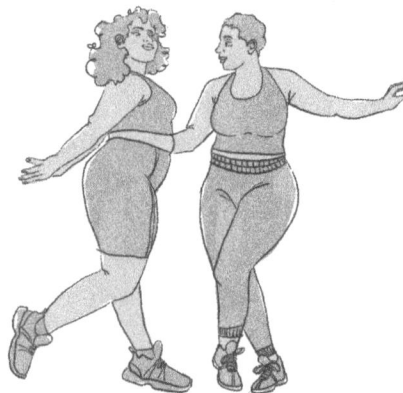

7) **Running.** Run laps around your space. Continue for **1 minute**.

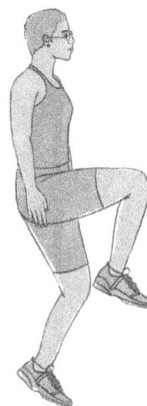

8) **Prayer.** Sit in Easy Pose and raise both arms straight overhead. Make a personal prayer or a wish for the day for **1 minute**.

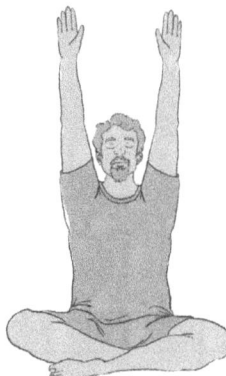

(4) Energizing Movement Fusion

June 16, 1993

There are no pauses between exercises unless indicated.

1) **Moving Arm Circles.** Stand straight with the feet shoulder-width apart. Bring the arms straight forward at shoulder level with the palms facing down. Make small, slow, outward circles with both arms. Keep circling and gradually moving faster as you raise the arms. When the arms are straight up, lean back from the hips. Hold this position for **10 seconds** with fast, strong circles. Still circling, bring the arms back to the starting position. Continue the motion, keeping the arms straight, for **4 minutes**.

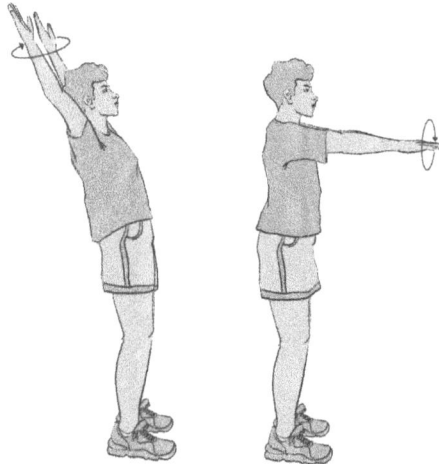

2) **Alternate Arm Reaches.** Remain standing with the feet shoulder-width apart. Bend forward from the hips to a 45-degree angle. Alternately stretch each arm forward with the palm facing down and bring it back, pushing the bent elbow back. Continue to move quickly (two arm movements per second) for **1 ½ minutes**.

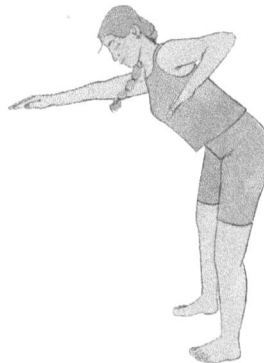

3) **Jump, Click the Heels, and Clap.** Remain standing, jump up, and simultaneously click the heels and clap the hands. The hands clap and the heels touch at the same time. Jump in rhythm for **3 ½ minutes**. (In the original class, Punjabi Drums were played to keep the rhythm.)

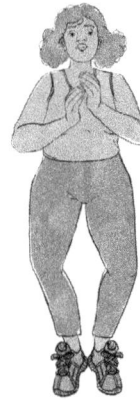

4) **Partner Wrestle.** ▲ Choose a partner and begin to wrestle. Try to take the other person down and pin them to the ground. Continue for **1 ½ minutes**.

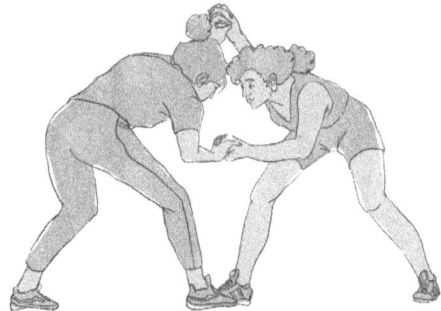

5) **Navel Pumps.** a) Sit in Easy Pose with a light Neck Lock and the left forearm balanced on top of the right forearm at shoulder level. Gaze straight ahead and pull the diaphragm up. Pump the navel in rhythm for **3 ½ minutes**. b) Relax the hands in the lap and chant **HAR** in rhythm (one repetition per second) for **1 ½ minutes**.

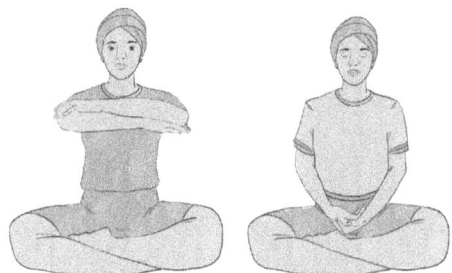

continue on next page »

6) **Bhangra Dance.** Stand up and dance to the music. Keep the arms raised above the Heart Center, move the shoulders up and down, and shift the weight from one foot to the other so that one foot is always off the ground. Continue for **5 ½ minutes**. Relax. (In the original class, Bhangra and Western electronic music were played.) *If doing this exercise in a group setting, dance with a partner.*

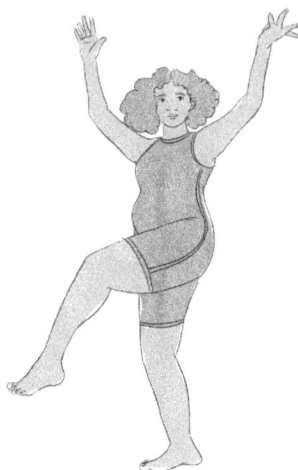

7) **People of Love.** Sit in Easy Pose with a straight spine and a light Neck Lock. Raise both arms straight overhead with the palms facing forward. Sing "We Are the People of Love" for **12 minutes**.

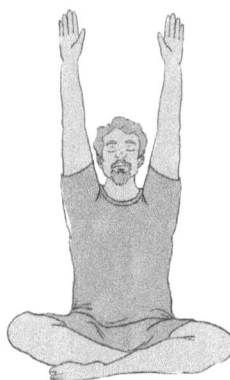

8) **Partner Wrestle.** ▲ Choose a partner and begin to wrestle. Try to take the other person down and pin them to the ground. Continue for **30 seconds**.

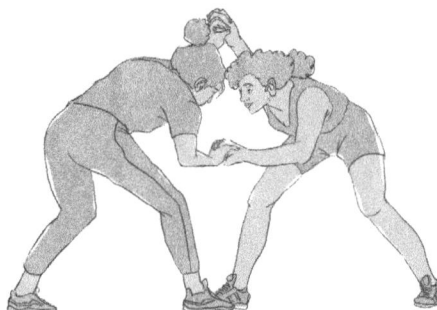

⑤ Stimulate the Kidneys and Control Your Total Being

June 17, 1993

There are no breaks between exercises unless indicated.

1) **Tree Pose Forward Bends.** Stand in Tree Pose and bring the right foot into the crease of the left hip, with the heel pressing the pubic bone. Balance and bend forward from the hips. Touch the ground in front of you with both hands and come back up. Count loudly: 1 down and 2 coming up. Continue for **2 minutes**. (In the original class, Punjabi Drums were played to keep the rhythm.) *Keep trying, no matter how many times you lose your balance. If practicing at sunrise, face the sun.*

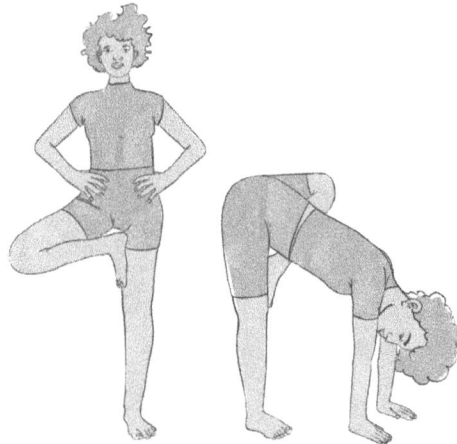

2) **Jump and Kick.** a) Stand with the hands on the hips. Hop onto your right leg and kick the left leg up and out to the side. Immediately hop onto the left leg and kick the right leg up and out (1 second per kick). Continuing to alternately kick the legs while hopping from one foot to the other for **2 minutes**.

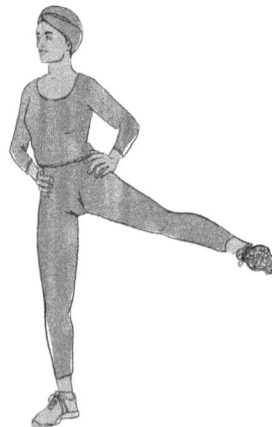

b) Keep the movement going and talk out loud to yourself for **2 minutes**. Relax.
If doing this exercise in a group setting, face a partner and talk to your partner.

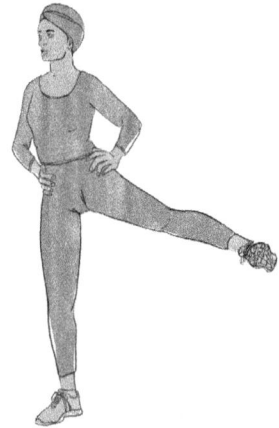

3) **Jump and Hit Chest and Thighs.** Stand and jump up, bending your knees and bringing the heels towards the buttocks. As you jump up, slap your chest with both hands, and as you land on the ground, slap the tops of the thighs. Jump at a fast pace (2 seconds per cycle) for **1 minute**.

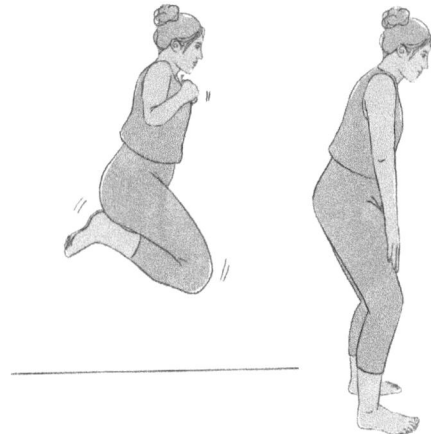

4) **Stimulate the Kidneys.** Remain standing. Hit the kidney area of the lower back alternately. Hit fast and hard. Keep the body straight; do not bend forward. Continue for **1 minute**. *This quickly circulates the blood in that area.*

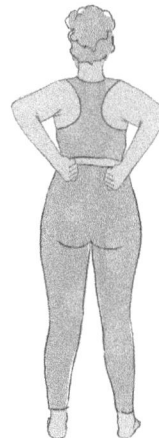

continue on next page »

5) **Meditation to Control Your Total Being**. a) Sit in Easy Pose with a straight spine and a light Neck Lock. Close the eyes. Meditate and chant **WAAH YANTEE**. Continue for **6 minutes**. b) Concentrate on sitting lightly and controlling your personal, mental, and spiritual being. Go into self-hypnosis: Sit light, be light. Continue for **1 minute**. c) Meditate and chant **WHAA-HAY GUROO WHAA-HAY JEEO** for **2 ½ minutes**. TO END: Inhale, suspend the breath, and squeeze the energy from the toes to the top of the head. Canon Fire exhale. Inhale deeply, suspend the breath, control the total self, and let it go. Inhale, suspend the breath, control the self, and let it go.

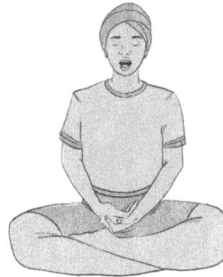

(6) Finding Balance through the Strength of the Spine

June 18, 1993

There are no breaks between exercises unless indicated.

1) **One-Leg Balance with Arm Circle.** a) Stand straight and raise the right arm up, palm facing forward. Bring the left knee up to the chest and hold it with the left hand. Balance for **1 ½ minutes.** b) Remain in the posture and make a fist with the right hand. Keep the right arm straight and move it in large backward circles as fast as possible. Continue for **2 minutes.** c) Switch sides and continue for **1 minute.** *This exercise helps to balance the hemispheres of the brain.*

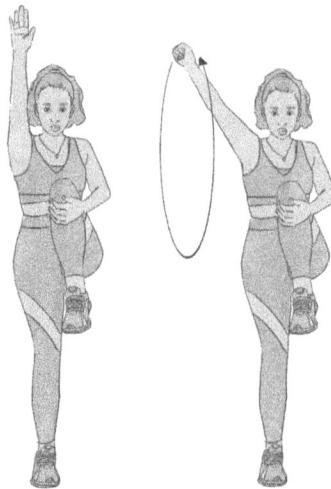

2) **Triangle Pose with Leg and Arm Extension.** a) Come into Triangle Pose with the feet wider than the shoulders. Keep the legs and arms straight, and press the heels into the ground. Focus on balancing the weight evenly

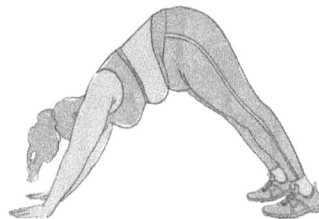

between the hands and the feet for
1 ½ minutes. b) Remain in the posture
and raise the right arm and left leg.
Balance for **1 minute**. c) Switch sides
and continue for **1 minute**. Relax.

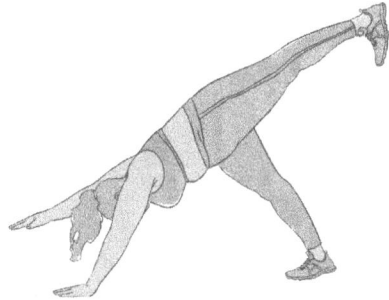

3) **Jog In Place.** Stand straight, and
with the hands in fists, jog in place.
Alternately swing each arm up to
shoulder level as you raise the opposite
knee to hip level. Keep the arms and
spine straight. Concentrate on the spine
and move with force for **5 minutes**.
Relax. (In the original class, Punjabi
Drums were played to keep the rhythm.)

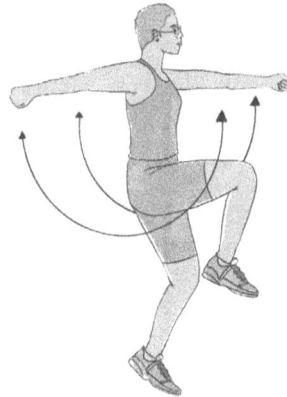

4) **Meditation Series With Kaal
Akaal.** a) Sit in Easy Pose with a
straight spine and a light Neck Lock.
Close the eyes. Sit lightly, lifting the
body upward from the abdomen so that
the weight is lighter on the sit bones.
Focus on controlling the flow of your
energy with the mind. Meditate for
3 minutes. b) Maintain the posture and
chant from the navel: **KAAL AKAAL,
SIREE AKAAL, MAHA AKAAL,
AKAAL MOORAT, WHA-HAY
GUROO.** Continue for **2 minutes**.

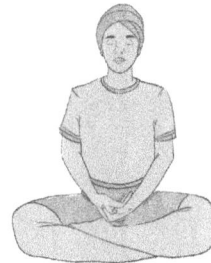

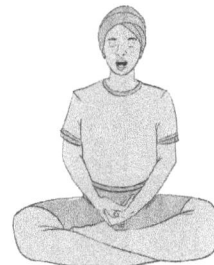

TO END: Raise both arms up over the head, palms facing forward, fingers spread wide. Feel the energy flow through all five fingers and try to control that flow of energy. Continue for **30 seconds**. Keep the arms up and extend the legs straight out in front, with the feet comfortably spread apart. Sit balanced with a straight spine and feel the energy in your toes. Continue for **30 seconds**. Relax.

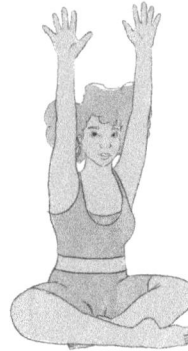

⑦ Core Strengthening and Spinal Flexibility Circuit

June 19, 1993

There are no breaks between exercises unless indicated.

1) **Triangle Pose Variation 1.** Come into Triangle Pose with the feet slightly wider than the hips and hands shoulder-width apart. Put all the weight on the hands; spread the fingers wide for increased strength and stability. Press the heels into the ground and keep the legs and arms straight. Continue for **3 ½ minutes**. *This stretch works on the sciatic nerve.*

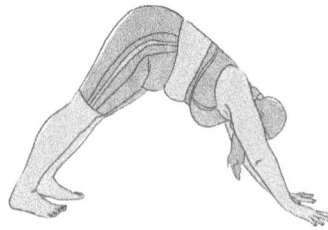

2) **Horse Kicks.** Maintain the position and bring the feet together. Kick both legs as high and hard as you can. Continue at a moderate pace (1 kick every 3 seconds) for **3 minutes**. Relax. *This exercise develops the central muscles of the lower spine.*

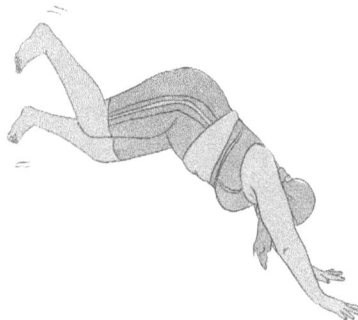

3) **Triangle Pose Variation 2**. Come into Triangle Pose. Balance the weight primarily on the hands, with the fingers spread wide. Put the feet together and press the heels into the ground to stretch the sciatic nerve. Keep the legs and arms straight. Hold the position for **1 minute**.

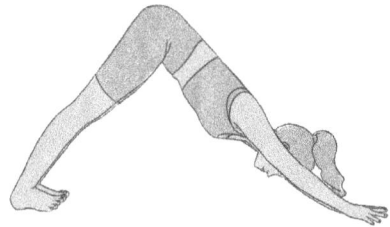

4) **Horse Kicks**. Maintain the position and kick both legs as high and hard as you can. Continue at a moderate pace (1 kick every 3 seconds) for **1 minute**.

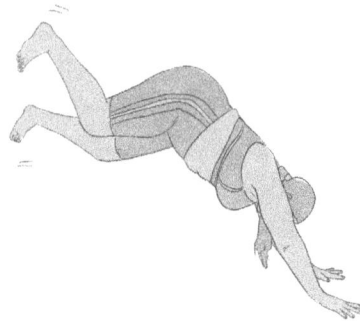

5) **Backward Stretch.** Stand straight with the feet shoulder-width apart. Extend the arms straight up overhead. Bend back from the hips and stretch the spine with very little pressure. Hold for **1 minute**.

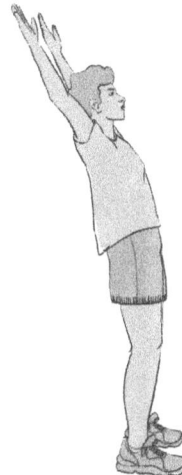

continue on next page »

6) **Parallel Forward Bend.** Remain standing with the feet shoulder-width apart. Extend the arms straight out in front of you, parallel to the ground. Slowly bend forward from the hips, keep the spine straight, and stretch forward until the upper body and arms are parallel to the ground. Hold for **30 seconds**. Relax.

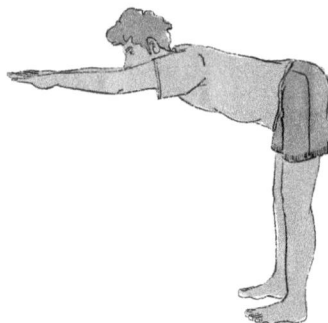

7) **Shake the Hips.** a) Stand straight with the feet shoulder-width apart. Bring the arms up to the sides, parallel to the ground, palms facing down, and elbows bent. Move the hips from side to side. Keep the arms and shoulders relaxed, the knees straight but not locked, and isolate the movement to the hips. Continue for **3 minutes**. b) Continue moving in rhythm for **8 ½ minutes**. (In the original class, Punjabi Drums were played to keep the rhythm.) *This exercise helps the liver release toxins.*

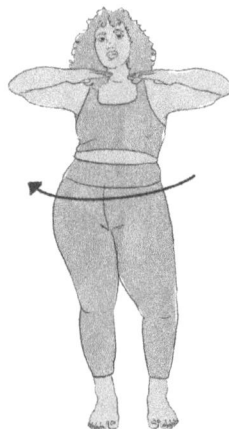

8) **Horse Kicks.** Come into Triangle Pose. Kick both legs as high and hard as you can. Continue at a moderate pace (1 kick every 3 seconds) for **1 minute**. Relax.

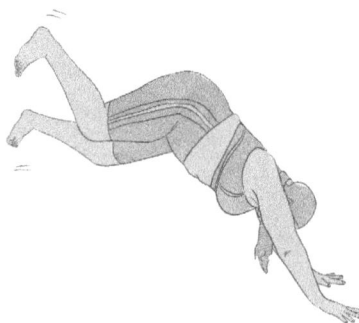

9) **Partner Wrestle.** ▲ Choose a partner and begin to wrestle. Try to take the other person down and pin them to the ground. Continue for **2 minutes**. Relax.

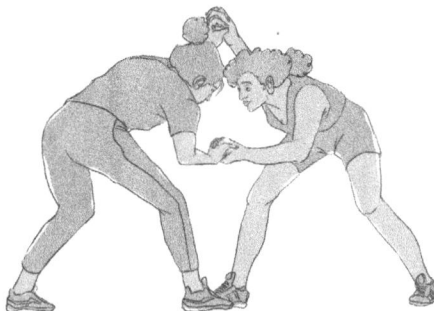

10) **Balance the Positive and Negative.** a) Sit in Easy Pose with a straight spine and a light Neck Lock. Raise both arms straight overhead, palms forward, and fingers spread wide. Balance the two sides of your body. Sit lightly; the pelvis is weightless. Sing "Happiness Runs in a Circular Motion" by Donovan from the Navel Point for **1 minute**. b) Meditate in the posture, concentrating on the navel, for **3 minutes**.

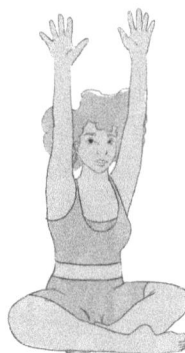

11) **Bowing Jaap Sahib**. Maintain the posture and sit still as you listen to the introduction. When the first Pauri begins, bow from the waist and bring the body and arms to the ground. Bow down with the first word of each line and come back up on the next word. Pause in the up position during the breaks in the recitation. Continue for **3 ½ minutes**.

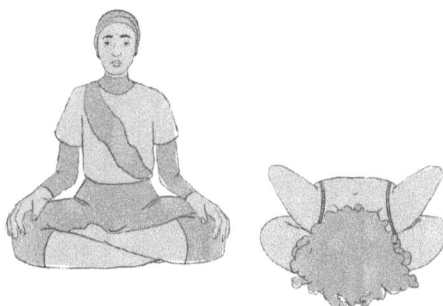

(8) Rhythmic Movements for Balance and Harmony

June 20, 1993

There are no breaks between exercises.

1) **One-Leg Balance.** Stand and, keeping both legs straight, raise the right leg back. Bring the left arm straight forward and the right arm alongside the body. With all the weight on the left leg, lean forward and allow the body to balance, creating a straight line from the toes to the fingertips. Continue for **3 ½ minutes**. Switch sides and continue for **1 ½ minutes**. Switch sides again and support the body on the heel of the left foot for **1 minute**. Switch sides and support yourself on the right heel for **30 seconds**.

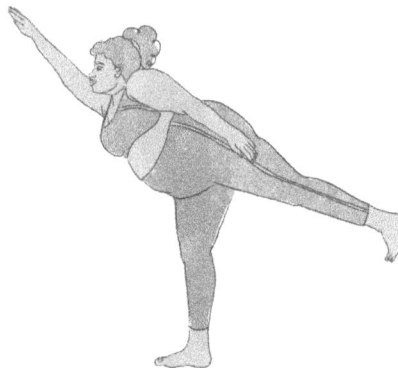

2) **Triangle Pose With Lower Back Massage.** Come into Triangle Pose with the feet flat and fingers separated. Keep the legs straight and the heels on the ground. Raise the right hand and hit the lower spine between the kidneys. Continue for **1 ½ minutes**. Switch hands and continue to hit with the left hand for **30 seconds**.

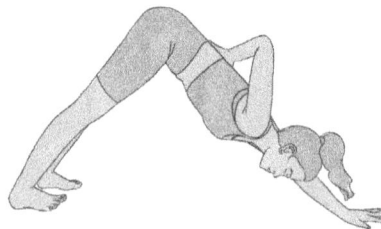

3) **Stimulate the Meridians.** Stand straight and, with both hands, hit the thighs as hard and fast as you can. Continue for **30 seconds**. Hit the groin area with fists for **30 seconds**. Hit the buttocks for **30 seconds**.

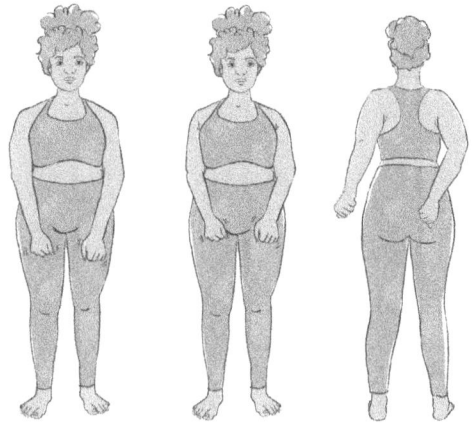

4) **Balance the Meridians.** Remain standing and raise the arms up. Bend the elbows and hit both ears with the palms, then bring them back up. Breathe in rhythm with the movement. Move rapidly, working up to Breath of Fire with the motion. Continue for **2 minutes**. *Listen to the sound that the hands make. All meridians meet in the ear, and when hit properly, they stimulate the entire body, balancing your energy.*

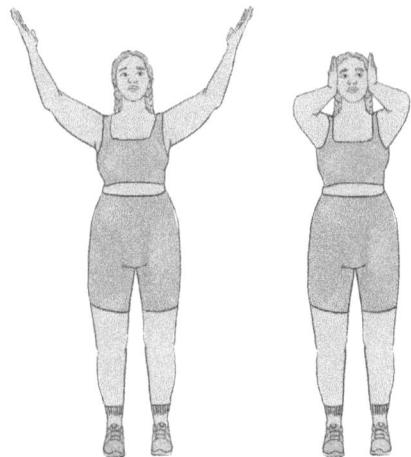

5) **Standing Torso Twist.** Remain standing and press the palms on the ears with the elbows open to the sides. Twist the body from side to side to the beat of the drum. Move rapidly (1 second per cycle) for **1 ½ minutes**. (In the original class, Punjabi Drums were played to keep the rhythm.)

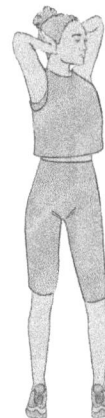

continue on next page »

6) **Standing Forward Bends With Hip Press.** Remain standing and interlock the hands against the back for balance. Bend forward from the hips and come back up, pressing the hips forward. Keep the spine and legs straight. Continue at a fast pace (1-2 seconds per cycle) for **2 minutes**. (In the original class, Punjabi Drums were played to keep the rhythm.) *The thigh muscle relates to the pituitary. If it is not developed, the pituitary does not function properly.*

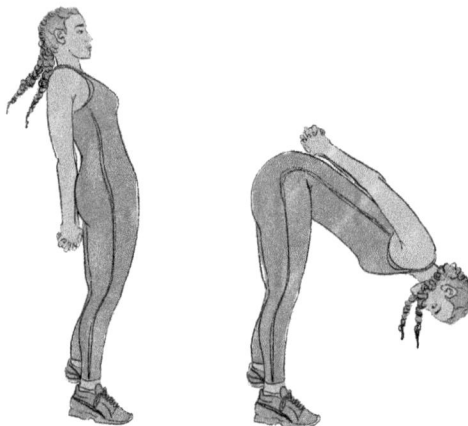

7) **Jump and Click the Heels.** Remain standing and hold the sides of the body just above the hip bones with both hands, elbows out to the sides. Jump up quickly and bring the heels together, then land on the balls of the feet. Continue at a fast pace (2 jumps per second) for **2 minutes**. (In the original class, Punjabi Drums were played to keep the rhythm.)

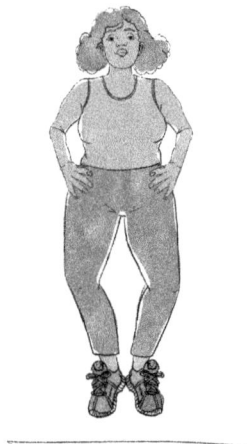

8) **Shake the Knees.** Remain standing and interlock the fingers behind the neck with the elbows out to the sides. Bend the knees slightly and begin to shake the knees in a fast, loose movement. Continue for **2 minutes**.

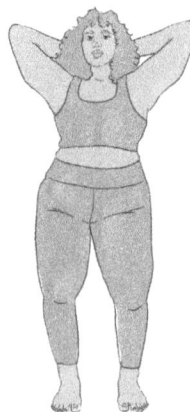

9) Shake the Hands and Knees.
Remain standing and bring the hands by the shoulders, palms facing forward. Rapidly shake the knees and hands. Create a heavy shiver that shakes the entire body. Continue for **1 minute**. *This exercise adjusts all the meridians of the body.*

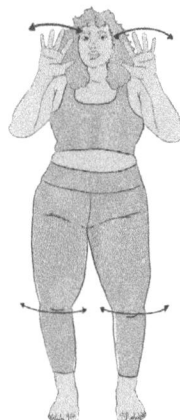

10) Sit and Stand. Stand up straight with the arms straight forward, cross the ankles, and sit down in Easy Pose. Stand up again without using the hands for support. Alternate between standing and sitting. Use the subtle energy in the hands to support the movement instead of physical strength. Consciously control the movement for **2 minutes**.

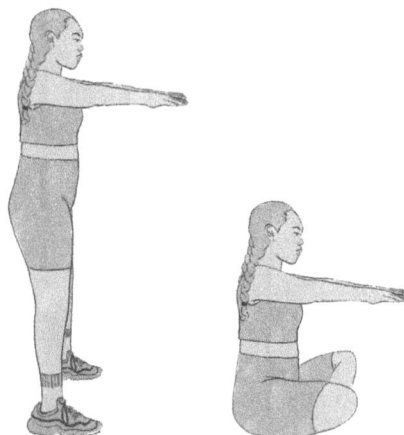

11) Meditation Series With Waah Yantee. a) Sit in Easy Pose with a straight spine and a light Neck Lock. Engage the Navel Point, eyes 1/10th open, and focus at the Tip of the Nose. Meditate for **2 minutes**. b) Maintain the posture and chant **WAAH YANTEE KAAR YANTEE** from the navel. Keep the navel center under your control. Continue for

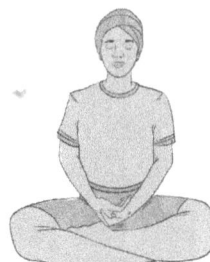

continue on next page »

3 minutes. (In the original class, the recording by Nirinjan Kaur was played.) c) Bring both hands to the shoulders with the fingers in front, thumbs in back, elbows out to the sides, and upper arms parallel to the ground. Continue chanting from the navel for **1 minute**. d) Interlace the fingers together, palms facing down, and bring the arms in an arc 6–8 inches above the head. Continue chanting from the navel for **1 minute**.

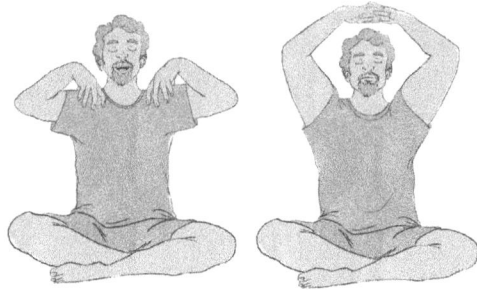

12) **Partner Wrestle.** ▲ Choose a partner and begin to wrestle. Try to take the other person down and pin them to the ground. Continue for **1 minute**.

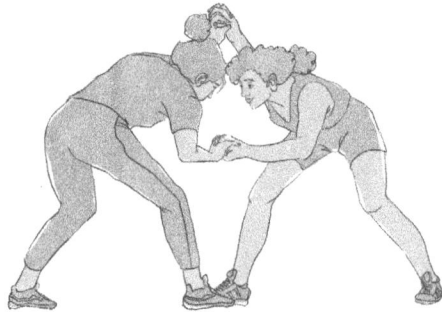

13) **Kick Dance.** a) Place the hands on the hips and kick alternate legs out to a 45-degree angle and parallel to the ground. Continue vigorously (1-2 cycles per second) for **2 ½ minutes**. (In the original class, Punjabi Drums were played to keep the rhythm.) b) Continue in rhythm with the music. Chant **HUMEE HUM BRAHM HUM** from the navel for **2 ½ minutes**. (In the original class, the recording "Humee Hum Brahm

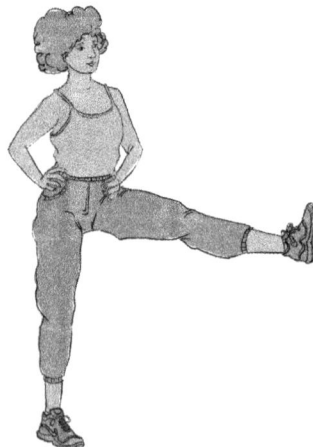

Hum" by Nirinjan Kaur was played.)
If doing this exercise in a group,
lock elbows with the people on both
sides, creating a line of energy.

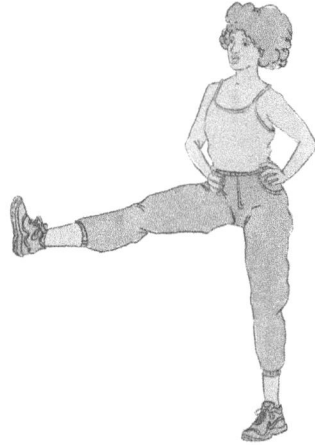

14) **Sit and Stand.** Stand up straight,
cross the ankles, and sit down in Easy
Pose. Stand up again without using
the hands for support. Alternate
between standing and sitting. Use
the subtle energy in the hands to
support the movement instead of
physical strength. Continue at a
medium pace for **2 ½ minutes**.
If doing this exercise in a class setting,
the teacher instructs the students to sit
and stand at random intervals. This trains
the physical body to respond quickly.

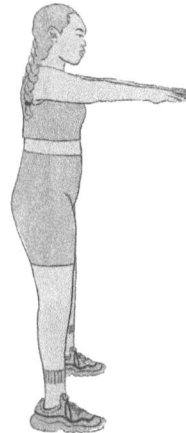

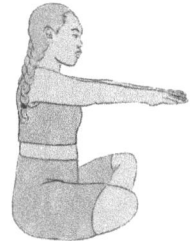

15) **Baby Pose.** Sit on your heels
in Rock Pose. Bend forward from
the hips and place the forehead
on the ground. Arms are at the
sides, palms facing up. Relax for **1
minute**. Remain in the posture and
chant **ONG NAMO GURU DEV
NAMO** loudly for **1 ½ minutes**.
(In the original class, the recording
by Nirinjan Kaur was played.)

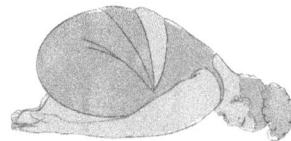

9 Stretch, Strengthen, and Revitalize

June 21, 1993

There are no breaks between exercises unless indicated.

1) **Navel Concentration.** a) Stand straight with the heels together and the feet open at a 45-degree angle. Keep the legs and spine straight. Put the hands on the hips, stand still, and concentrate on the Navel Point and hips. Mentally pull that area up and make it lighter and weightless. Continue for **2 ½ minutes**. b) Remain in this posture and bend back 40 degrees from the hips. Continue concentrating on the navel and hips for **2 minutes**. Come up slowly.

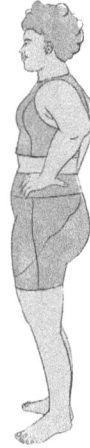

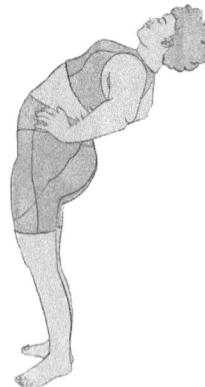

2) **Aura Adjustment Series.** a) Stand straight with the heels together and the feet open at a 45-degree angle. Raise the arms out to the sides and up to 60 degrees with the palms facing down. Tense the fingers and spread them as wide as possible. Close your eyes and hold for **1 minute**. b) Remain in the posture and bend forward from the hips to 45 degrees. Hold for **1 minute**, keeping tension and strength in the fingers. c) Remain in the posture and drop the arms. Relax the neck and shoulders, and let the arms hang loose. Keep the neck and spine straight. Hold calmly for **1 minute**. d) Remain in this posture with loose arms and shoulders, balance on the right foot, and slowly raise the left leg back. Continue for **3 minutes**. e) Switch sides and balance for **1 ½ minutes**. *Allow the body to shake, and the mind and spirit will come to help.*

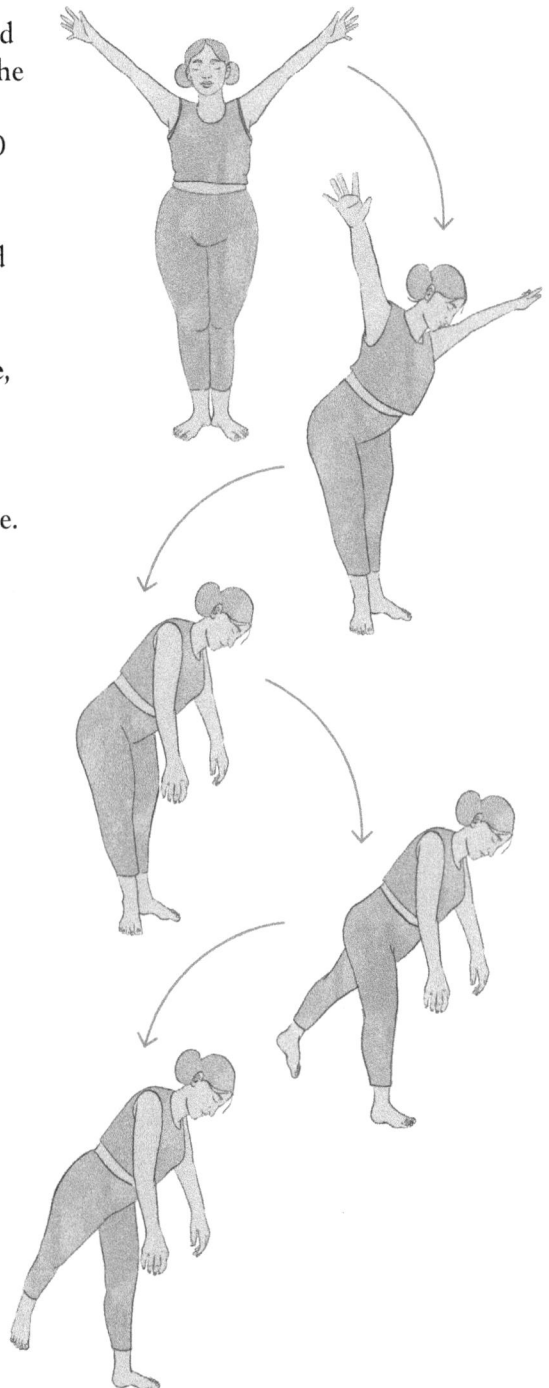

continue on next page »

3) **Life Nerve Stretch Variation.**
a) Stand with the legs spread as wide apart as possible. Interlace the fingers with palms facing up and stretch the arms up straight. Hold steady for **3 minutes**. b) Slowly bend forward from the hips and bring the arms between the legs. Release the hands and hold the sit bones. Continue for **2 minutes**. TO END: Slowly rise up to the starting posture with interlaced hands. Bring the legs together and stretch the arms up for **30 seconds**.

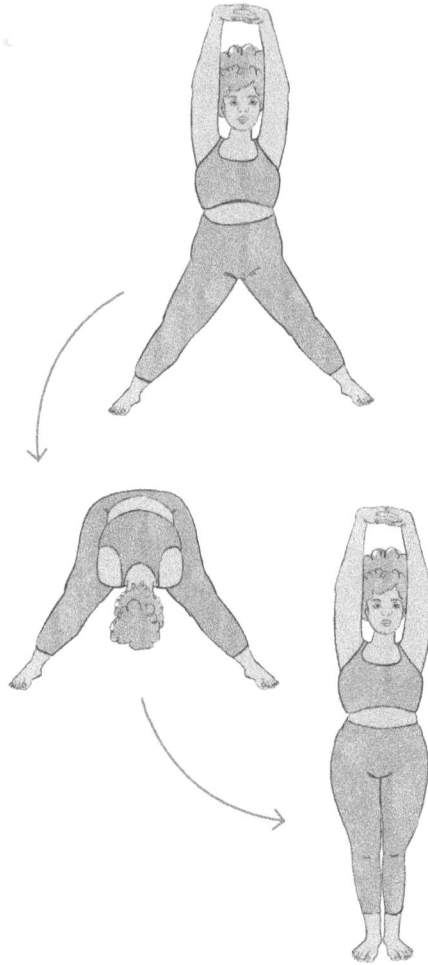

4) **Hit the Chest.** Sit on the heels in Rock Pose with the knees spread wide. Make fists with both hands and hit the chest as fast and powerfully as you can. Continue for **3 minutes**. (In the original class, Bhangra music was played to keep the rhythm.) Relax.

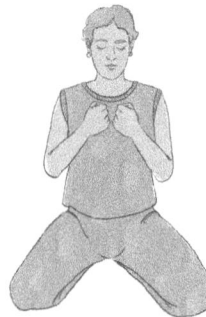

74

5) **Circle Clap.** Remain sitting in Rock Pose with the knees spread wide. Clap the hands in front of the upper body. Then circle the arms up and out, coming back to clap again, creating a 36-inch (91 cm) diameter circle. Continue rapidly and let the body create its own ecstatic dance for **3 ½ minutes**. (In the original class, Punjabi Drums were played to keep the rhythm.) *This exercise calms the nervous system.*

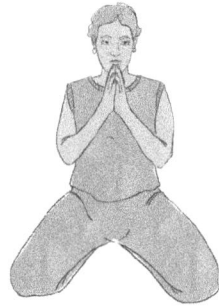

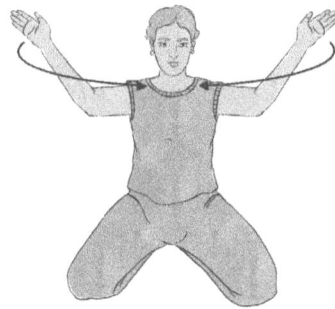

6) **Sit in the Sun.** Sit in Easy Pose with a straight spine and a light Neck Lock facing the sun. Relax the elbows by the sides, bring the forearms up, and angle the palms toward the sun. Close the eyes and let the sun shine on the eyelids and forehead. Pump the Navel Point as fast as you can without coordinating with the breath. Continue for **4 minutes**. b) Remain in the posture, continue to pump the Navel Point, and chant **WAAH YANTEE KAAR YANTEE** for **3 minutes**. (In the original class, the recording by Nirinjan Kaur was played.) Relax.

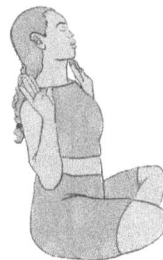

⑩ Flexibility and Vigor Unleashed

June 25, 1993

There are no breaks between exercises unless indicated.

1) **Propeller Arms.** Stand with the feet wider than shoulder-width apart. Make fists and circle the arms in opposite directions (one arm circling forward and the other circling backward). Keep the arms straight and move from the shoulders rapidly (2 circles per second) for **2 minutes**.

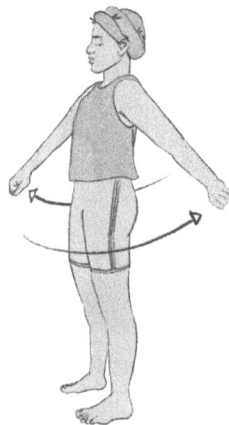

2) **Hop Kicks** a) Stand with the feet shoulder-width apart and the hands on the hips. Hop onto one leg while kicking the other leg forward and up. Continue alternately kicking the legs for **1 minute**. b) Sing with the movement for **1 minute**. (In the original class, "Happiness Runs in a Circular Motion" by Donovan was sung.)

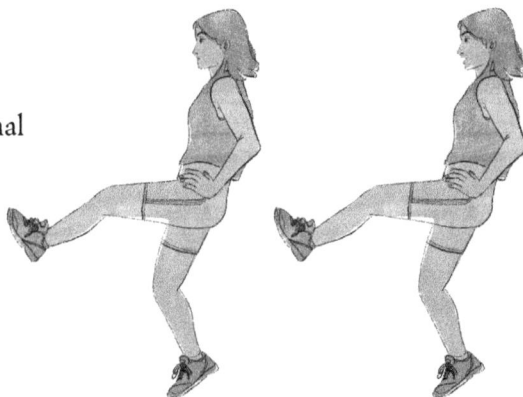

3) Propeller Arms and Hop Kicks.
Combine exercises 1 and 2. Make
fists with your hands and circle
the arms in opposite directions
as you hop on alternate legs and
kick. Continue for **2 minutes**.

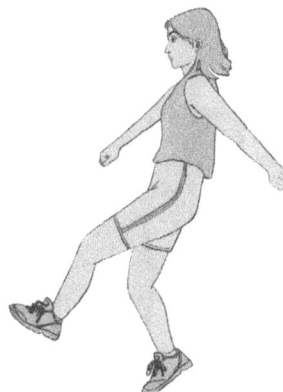

**4) Parallel Forward Bend Heels
Together.** Stand straight with the
heels together and the toes open at
a 45-degree angle. Stretch the arms
straight forward, palms facing down.
Bend from the hips and stretch
forward so the upper body and arms
are parallel to the ground. Keep the
legs and spine straight. Hold for **4
½ minutes**. Come up very slowly.
*This exercise puts pressure on the
meridians relating to the digestive organs,
lymph glands, and brain. It is a good
posture to practice for 5 minutes daily.*

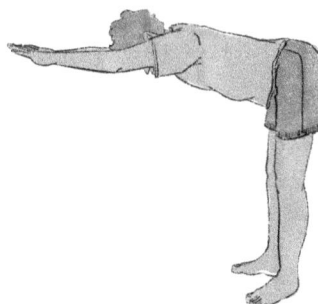

5) Hop on One Foot. Stand straight
and place the hands on the hips. Hop
up and down on one foot. Switch feet
as needed. Give equal time to both
legs. Continue for **3 ½ minutes**.
This exercise develops the thighs.

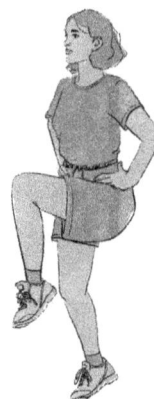

continue on next page »

6) **Standing Torso Rotation.**
Stand with the feet as wide apart
as possible. Place the hands on the
hips and rotate the torso in wide
circles in either direction. Keep
the legs straight and make full
circles. Continue for **4 minutes**.
*This exercise helps to remove built-
up waste in the digestive system.*

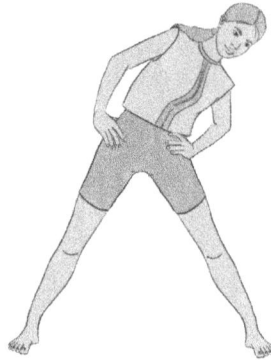

7) **Shoulder Shrugs.** Sit in Easy
Pose with a straight spine. Hold the
knees with the arms straight. Lift both
shoulders up towards the ears and
immediately drop them back down.
Move rapidly for **1 ½ minutes**.
*This motion helps circulate the blood
to the head and adjust the ribs.*

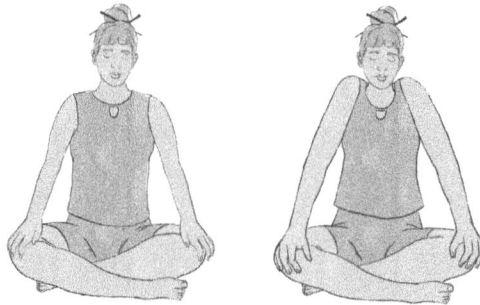

8) **Spinal Twists.** Remain in Easy
Pose and grasp the shoulders with
the fingers in front and the thumbs in
back. The upper arms are parallel to
the ground, and the elbows are out
to the sides. Twist the body rapidly
from side to side for **1 ½ minutes**.

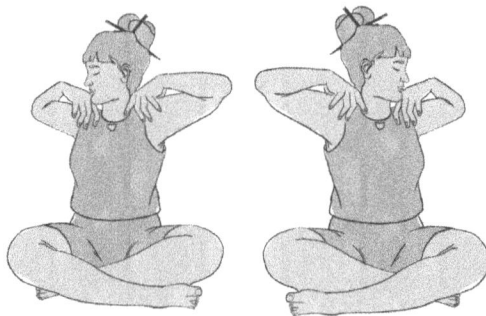

9) **Rope Pulls.** Sit in Easy Pose. Alternately reach forward as if grasping a rope, then make a fist and pull back towards the body. Draw the fists in powerfully for **1 minute**. Open the hand as it extends out and close it as if grasping a rope to pull it in. Move rapidly for **1 ½ minutes**.

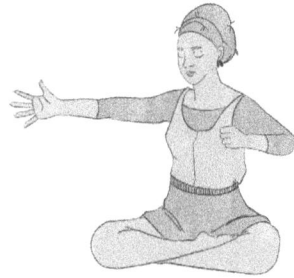

10) **Practice Pratyahar.** Sit in Easy Pose with a straight spine and a light Neck Lock. Place both hands on the Heart Center, one on top of the other. Close the eyes. a) Sit in a state of Pratyahar. Make your body and mind still. As thoughts come to your mind, don't engage with them. Continue for **2 ½ minutes**. b) Don't listen to the music. Refuse to participate and have no thoughts. Continue for **7 ½ minutes**. (In the original class, "Sat Siri, Siri Akal" by Nirinjan Kaur was played.) c) Chant with the music for **4 minutes**. Relax. (In the original class, "Sat Siri, Siri Akal" by Nirinjan Kaur was played.)

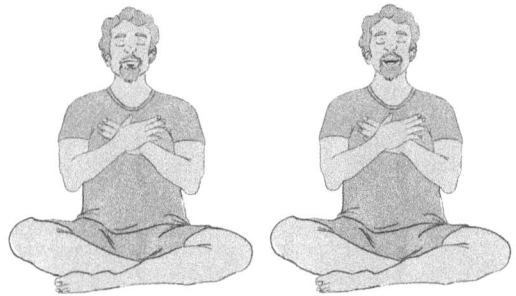

11) **Song of Bliss.** Remain in Easy Pose and sing with the music. Continue for **5 ½ minutes**. (In the original class, "I am Bountiful, Blissful, Beautiful" by Nirinjan Kaur from the Musical Affirmations Collection was played.)

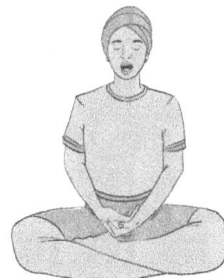

(11) Heartbeat Resonance Practice

June 28, 1993

There are no breaks between exercises unless indicated.

1) **Parallel Forward Bend.** Stand with the feet wider than the shoulders. Extend the arms straight up, palms forward. Bend from the hips until the torso and arms are parallel to the ground, with the fingers spread wide. The head is up, not in Neck Lock. Stretch forward with the arms and head and back with the hips. Create a balance, keeping the arms, legs, and spine straight. Continue for **5 ½ minutes**. *This exercise stretches the sciatic nerve and maintains rhythmic circulation.*

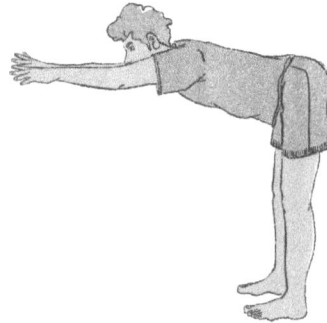

2) **Pelvic Balance.** Stand straight with the feet shoulder-width apart. Raise both arms in an arc over the head, with the tips of the Jupiter (index) and Saturn (middle) fingers touching. Fingers are spread wide, and palms face forward. Move the pelvis forward and back to the starting position. Isolate the movement to the pelvis. Keep the spine and knees straight.

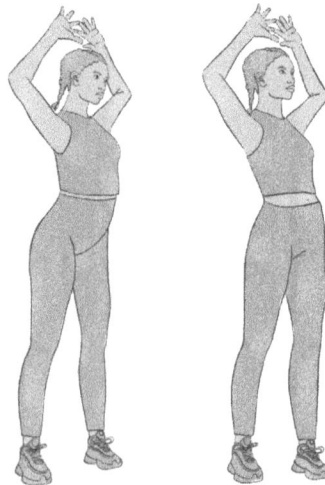

Move quickly (one cycle per second) for **4 minutes**. (In the original class, Punjabi Drums were played to keep the rhythm.) Stretch and relax.
This exercise works on the strength of the diaphragm and adjusts the pelvic area.

3) **Knee Bends with Arms Extended.**
a) Stand straight with the feet a little wider than the shoulders and the feet angled out. Extend both arms straight out to the sides, parallel to the ground, with the left palm facing down and right palm facing up. Bend the knees outward and move down about 18 inches (45 centimeters). Squeeze both hands into fists as you go down, opening them as you come up. Squeeze the fists tighter and tighter. Continue (one cycle per second) for **2 minutes**. b) Reverse the hand positions, left hand up and right hand down, and continue for **2 minutes**. (In the original class, Punjabi Drums were played to keep the rhythm.)
The knees and heart are related; this exercise works on the heart.

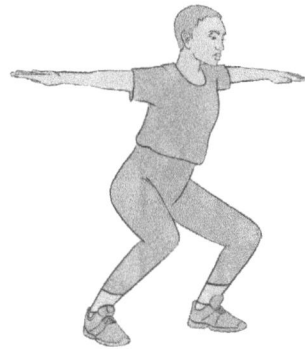

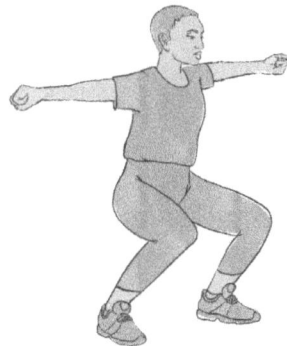

continue on next page »

4) **Jumping Jacks**. Stand straight with the arms at your sides. Jump and open the legs wide as you bring both arms straight up and clap the hands over the head (1 clap per second). Jump again and bring the feet together and the arms down to your sides. Continue alternately jumping from one position to the other in a continuous motion for **2 ½ minutes**. (In the original class, Punjabi Drums were played to keep the rhythm.)

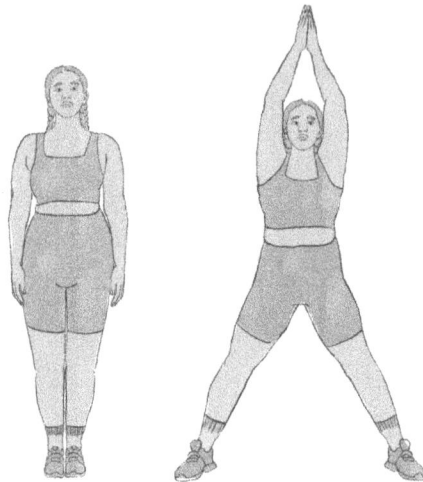

5) **Parallel Forward Bend.** Repeat Exercise 1. Hold for **3 minutes**.

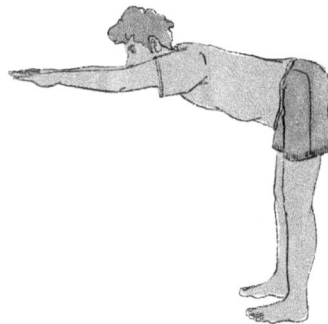

6) **Standing Circular Movement**. Stand with the feet shoulder-width apart. Raise the arms up parallel to each other. The elbows are relaxed and bent. Create a spiral movement with the entire body, from the tips of the toes to the hands. Continue for **2 minutes**. (In the original class, Punjabi Drums were played to keep the rhythm.) *Move the legs and arms similarly and create a balance.*

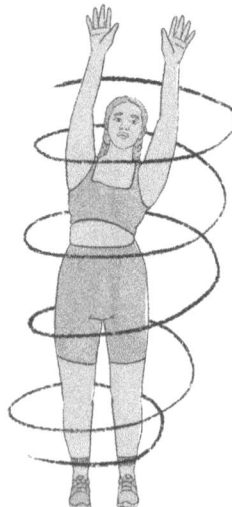

7) **Pelvic Balance.** Repeat Exercise 2. Continue for **1 minute**. (In the original class, Punjabi Drums were played to keep the rhythm.)

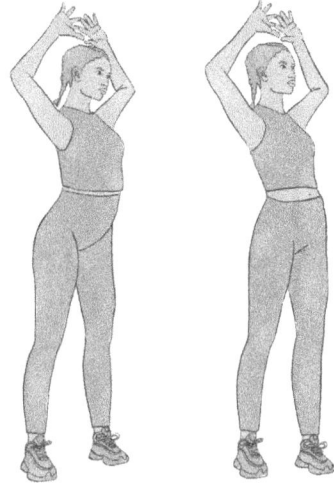

8) **Stand in the Sun.** a) Stand facing the rising sun with the feet shoulder-width apart. Raise both arms up, palms forward. Close the eyes and let the sun shine on your forehead, eyelids, and palms of the hands. Hold for **1 ½ minutes**. b) Turn around with your back to the sun. Keep the arms straight up and open the eyes wide. Look straight forward, gaze parallel to the ground, and imagine you are looking into the cosmic eye. Hold this position for **1 minute**. Relax. (In the original class, "Har Singh Nar Singh" by Nirinjan Kaur was played.)

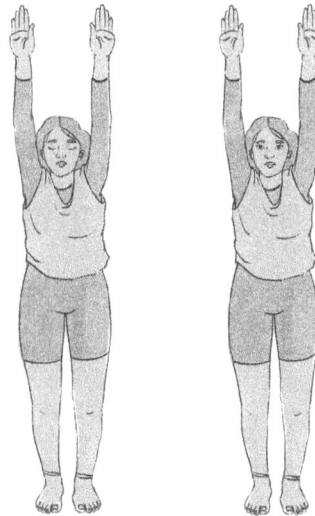

continue on next page »

9) **Shuniya Concentration.** a) Come sitting on the heels with the knees spread apart. Place the hands on the crease of the hips, with the fingers in front and the thumbs in back. Keep the spine straight and apply a light Neck Lock. Close the eyes and come into a state of *shuniya*—"I am nothing." Continue for **1 ½ minutes**. (In the original class, "Har Singh Nar Singh" by Nirinjan Kaur was played.)
b) Concentrate and bring all energy to the Navel Point. Mentally chant the mantra:

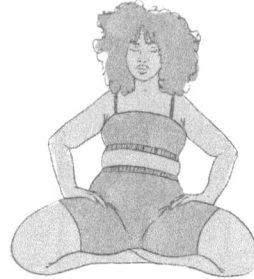

**WAAH YANTEE KAAR YANTEE JAGADOOTPATEE
AADAK IT WHAA-HAA
BRAHMAADAY
TRAYSHAA GUROO
IT WHAA-HAY GUROO**

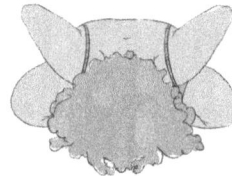

Continue for **4 minutes**. (In the original class, the recording by Nirinjan Kaur was played.) c) Keeping the hands in place, bend forward, relax the shoulders down, and rest the forehead on the ground. Sing with the music. Continue for **1 minute**.

10) **Bhangra Dance**. Stand up and dance to the beat. Keep the arms raised above the Heart Center, move the shoulders up and down, and shift the weight from one foot to the other so that one foot is always off the ground. Continue for **3 ½ minutes**.

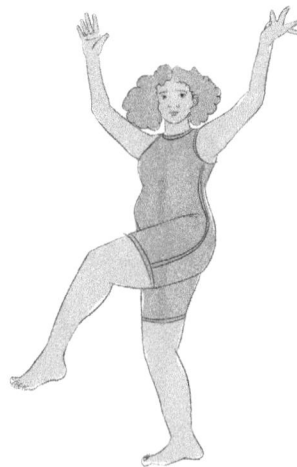

TO END: Sit in Easy Pose and laugh loudly for **30 seconds**. Scream as loudly as you can for **30 seconds**. (In the original class, Punjabi Drums were played to keep the rhythm.)

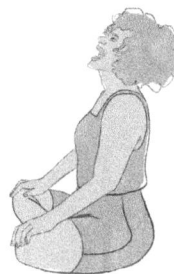

11) **Hit the Chest**. Remain in Easy Pose with a light Neck Lock. Make fists with both hands and begin to hit the chest as fast and powerfully as you can. Continue for **1 minute**. *Everyone experiences grief that is held in the chest; just beat it away.*

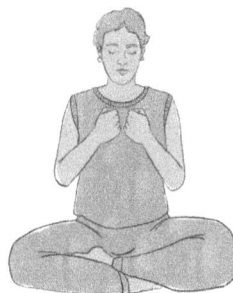

12) **People of Love.** Remain in Easy Pose with a light Neck Lock. Clap your hands (one clap per second) and sing "We Are the People of Love."[5] Continue for **2 minutes**.

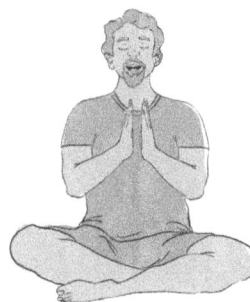

---

5   A version of this music by Avtar Singh Khalsa can be found on Gurbani Media Center at https://play.sikhnet.com/ You can also find a version by Snatam Kaur on Spotify by searching for "People of Love."

continue on next page »

13) **Self Healing**. Remain in Easy Pose. Gently touch any part of the body that needs healing. Continue for **2 minutes**. (In the original class, the recording "Heal Me" by Guru Shabad Singh was played.) *Use the energy that you have created now to heal yourself.*

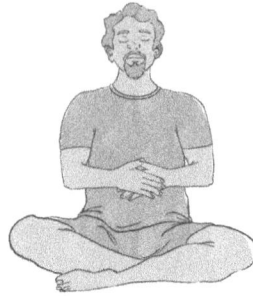

14) **Turtle Pose**. a) Lie down on the stomach with the chin on the ground. Extend the arms forward on the ground. Beat the ground with both arms and legs (move from the shoulders and hips). Continue for **1 minute**. b) Crawl forward like a turtle for **30 seconds**.

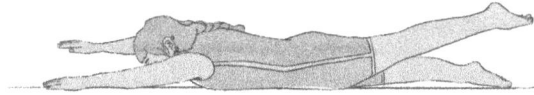

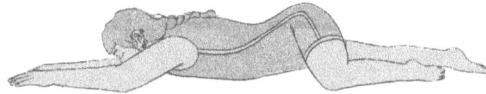

15) **Kick the Buttocks Hit the Chest.** a) Come lying down on your back, bend the knees up, kick the buttocks with the heels, and hit the chest with your fists. Move fast and use force for **30 seconds**. b) Continue to kick the buttocks and hit the navel area with your fists for **30 seconds**.

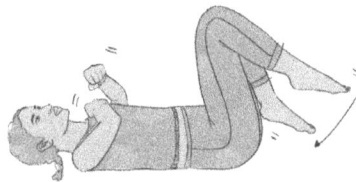

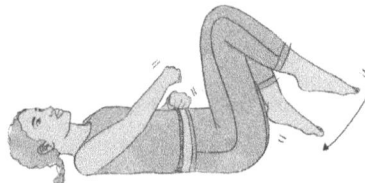

16) **Facial Circulation**. Sit in Easy Pose. Slap the face, neck, ears, and head with the hands to stimulate the flow of blood to these areas. Move fast for **1 minute**.
TO END: Use the Jupiter (index) fingers and thumbs to grasp the earlobes. Quickly pull down, release, and repeat. Continue for **15 seconds**.

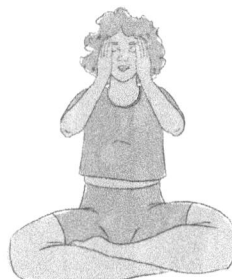

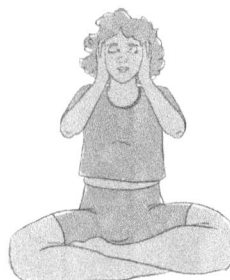

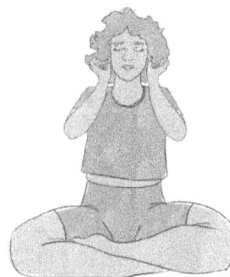

(12) Strengthening and Elevating Core Energy

June 29, 1993

There are no breaks between exercises unless indicated.

1) **Ostrich Dance.** Bend forward with palms on the ground and straight legs. Place equal weight on all four limbs, and move the pelvis from side to side in rhythm for **4 minutes**. (In the original class, Punjabi Drums were played to keep the rhythm.) Relax. *The pelvic triangle (from the hips to the Navel Point) is the source of human balance and strength.*

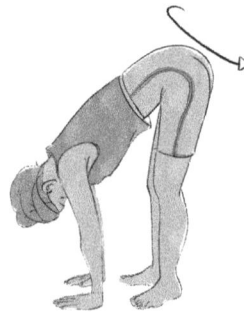

2) **Jumping Jacks.** Stand straight with the arms at your sides. Jump and open the legs wide as you bring both arms straight up and clap the hands over the head (1 clap per second). Jump again and bring the feet together and the arms down to your sides. Continue alternately jumping from one position to the other in a continuous motion for **3 minutes**. (In the original class, Punjabi Drums were played to keep the rhythm.)

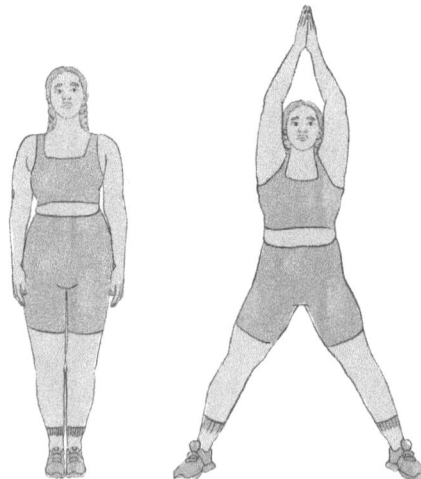

3) **Hip Bounce.** Lie on the stomach, chin on the ground, arms on the ground extended straight forward. Interlock the hands and point the toes. Using the stability of the arms, chest, and toes, raise the pelvis off the ground and drop it back down. Move quickly for **3 minutes**. (In the original class, Punjabi Drums were played to keep the rhythm.)

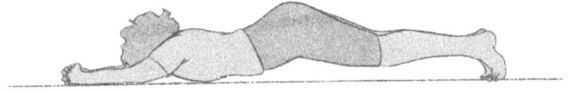

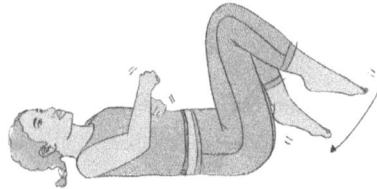

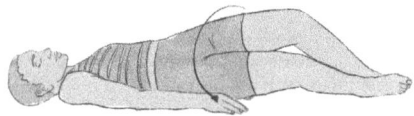

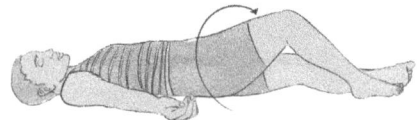

4) **Kick the Buttocks Hit the Stomach.** Turn onto the back and bend the knees, bringing the heels off the ground. Kick the buttocks with alternate heels and hit the stomach with alternate fists. Move fast with force for **1 minute**. (In the original class, Punjabi Drums were played to keep the rhythm.)

5) **Toss and Turn.** Lie on the back and press the shoulders into the ground. Keeping the head and shoulders stationary, twist and turn the rest of the body. Continue for **1 ½ minutes**. (In the original class, Punjabi Drums were played to keep the rhythm.)

continue on next page »

6) **Sat Kriya.** Sit in Rock Pose with the knees spread wide, the spine straight, and a light Neck Lock. Engage the Navel Point and root down to the Earth. Raise the arms straight up and interlace the fingers with the index fingers extended. (For working with masculine, projective energy, place the right thumb over the left. For working feminine, reflective energy, place the left thumb over the right.) Chant **SAT** and pull the Navel Point in and up. Chant **NAAM** as you release it. Keep the rib cage lifted and the shoulders down. Continue for **1 minute** (8 cycles per 10 seconds). Relax. (In the original class, Punjabi Drums were played to keep the rhythm.)

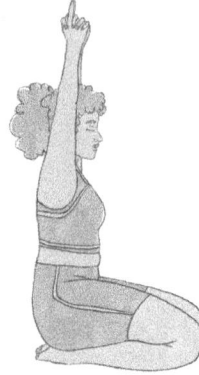

7) **Sat Kriya Bowing.** Maintain the posture. Inhale and pull the navel in as you say **SAT**. Keep the navel contracted and the breath held as you bend forward, touching the ground with the forehead. Exhale and release the navel as you say **NAM** and come back up (2 seconds per cycle). Continue for **2 ½ minutes**. Relax.

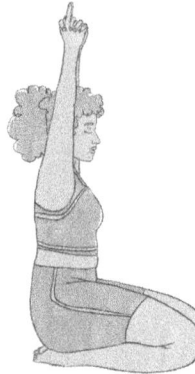

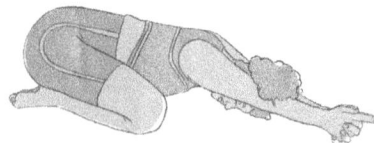

8) **Bowing Jaap Sahib.** Maintain the posture and hold still during the introduction. When the first Pauri begins, bend at the hips as you bring the forehead to touch the ground. Bow down with the first word of each line and come back up on the second word. Pause in the up position during the breaks in the recitation. Continue for **1 ½ minutes**. Relax.

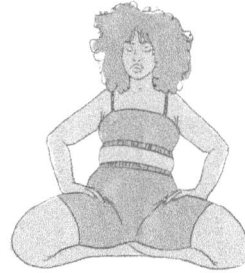

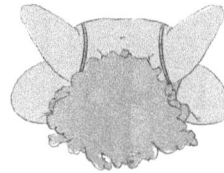

9) **Frog Pose Meditation.** Sit in Frog Pose with a straight spine and apply a light Neck Lock. Close the eyes and imagine the spine as a tube of light. Meditate in this posture for **3 ½ minutes**. (In the original class, "Meditation" by Wahe Guru Kaur was played.)

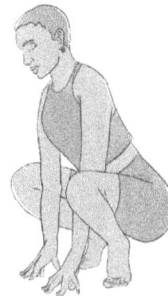

10) **Sit and Stand in the Sun.** Sit in Easy Pose with a straight spine and a light Neck Lock facing the sun. Relax the elbows by the sides, bring the forearms up, and angle the palms toward the sun. Close the eyes and let the sun shine on the eyelids and forehead. Drop all tension and completely relax. Hold for **1 ½ minutes**. Stand up and hold the posture for **30 seconds**.

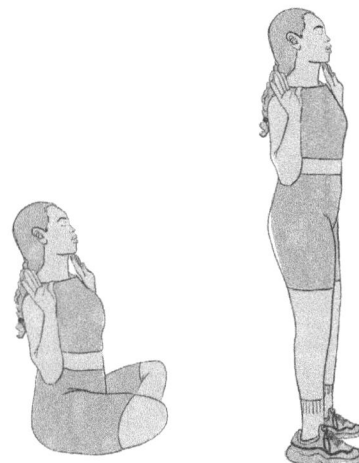

(13) Transformative Exercises for the Whole Body

June 30, 1993

There are no breaks between exercises unless indicated.

1) **Standing Balance Series.** Stand straight. a) Raise the left leg behind you and grasp the foot with both hands. Balance in this posture for **1 minute**. b) Release the right hand only, bend forward, and place it on the ground in front of you. Hold for **2 ½ minutes**. c) Stand up and change sides. Grasp the right foot with both hands and balance for **30 seconds**. d) Release the left hand only, bend forward, and place it on the ground in front of you. Hold for **1 minute**. *This exercise works on the reproductive glands.*

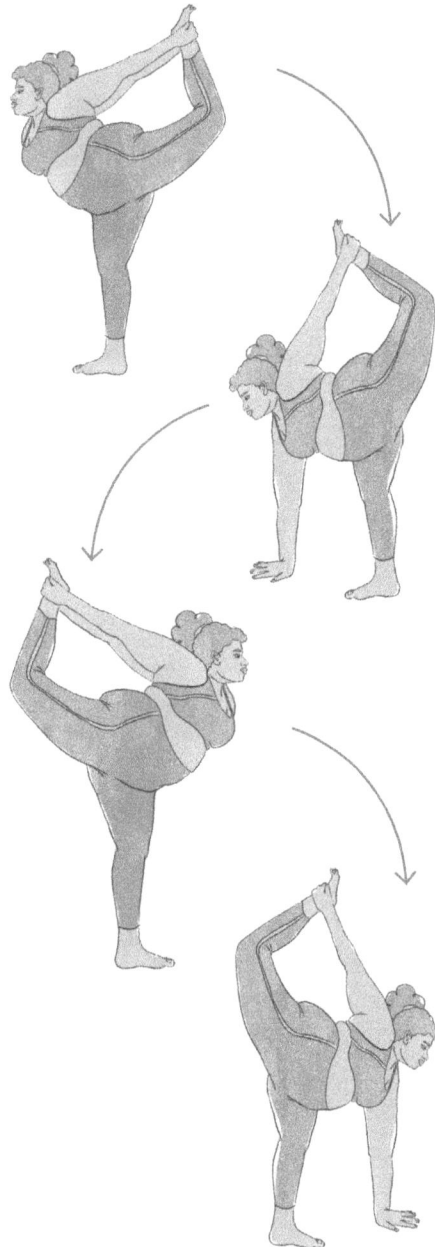

2) **Backwards Stretch Variation.** Stand straight with the heels together and the feet open to 45 degrees. Interlace the fingers behind the neck with the elbows out to the sides. Stretch backward from the pelvis to a 60-degree angle. Keep the legs straight. Hold and meditate on the heavens for **2 minutes**.

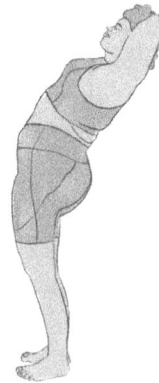

3) **Jumping Jacks.** Jump and open the legs wide as you bring both arms straight up and clap the hands over the head (1 clap per second). Jump again and bring the feet together and the arms down to your sides. Continue alternately jumping from one position to the other in a continuous motion for **5 minutes**. (In the original class, Punjabi Drums were played to keep the rhythm.) *This exercise stimulates the thyroid gland and builds stamina.*

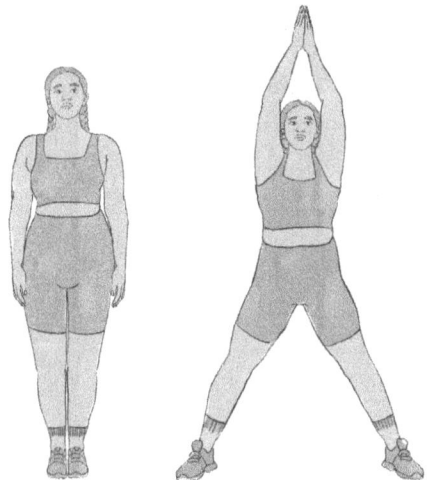

4) **Partner Wrestle.** ▲ Choose a partner, and begin to wrestle. Try to take the other person down and pin them to the ground. Continue for **1 minute**.

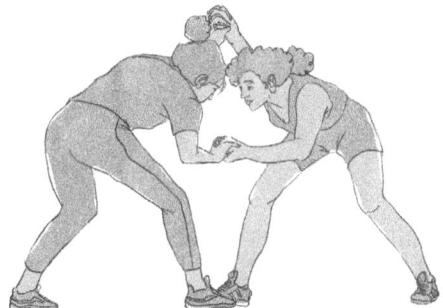

continue on next page »

5) **Frog Pose Clap.** Squat on with the heels together and off the ground and the fingertips on the ground between the knees, close to the body, in Frog Pose. Clap the hands together, then place them back on the ground. Keeping the fingertips on the ground, straighten the legs, raise the hips and bring the head down, then come back to the starting position. Continue this sequence for **2 ½ minutes**. (In the original class, Punjabi Drums were played to keep the rhythm.)

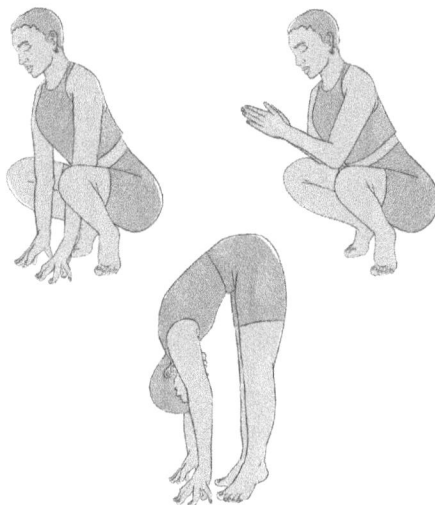

6) **Bhangra Dance.** Stand up and dance to the music. Keep the arms raised above the Heart Center, move the shoulders up and down, and shift the weight from one foot to the other so that one foot is always off the ground. Continue for **2 ½ minutes**. (In the original class, Bhangra music was played.)

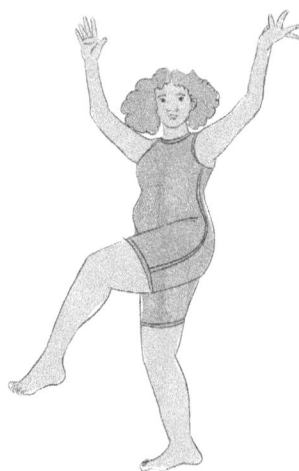

7) **Squats.** Stand straight with the feet shoulder-width apart. Squat down and come back up in a steady rhythm (2 seconds per cycle). Continue for **1 minute**. (In the original class, Punjabi Drums were played to keep the rhythm.) *If doing this exercise in a group, stand in line and hold hands with people on either side.*

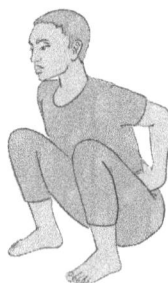

8) **Boat Pose Lifts.** Lie on your stomach, chin on the ground, with the arms extended straight forward, palms on the ground, legs straight, and heels together. Raise the arms, shoulders, head, and both legs and lower them down in a steady rhythm, chanting **HAR** as you lift up (2 seconds per cycle). Continue for **2 ½ minutes**. (In the original class, Punjabi Drums were played to keep the rhythm.)

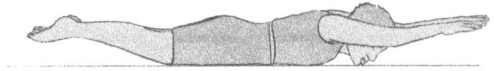

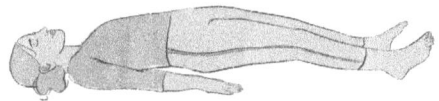

9) **Back Body Drops.** Lie on the back with the arms at the sides, palms facing down. Use the hands and heels to lift the body up and drop down in a steady rhythm, chanting **HAR** as you lift up (2 seconds per cycle). The head and shoulders remain on the ground. Continue for **1 ½ minutes**. (In the original class, Punjabi Drums were played to keep the rhythm.)

10) **Alternate Leg Lifts.** a) Remain on the back and place the palms face down. Alternately raise each leg to 90 degrees in a steady rhythm as you chant **HAR** from the navel and lower it. Keep the leg straight and chant **HAR** from the navel on the lift. Continue for **2 minutes**. b) Raise both legs together, chanting **HAR** as you lift up. Keep the legs straight. Continue for **30 seconds**. (In the original class, Punjabi Drums were played to keep the rhythm.)

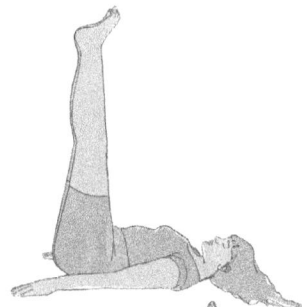

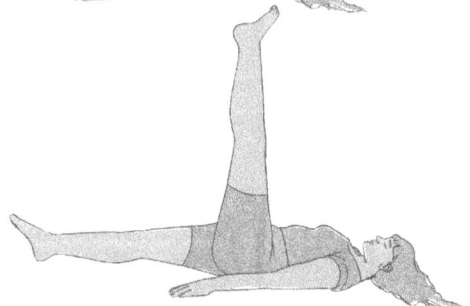

continue on next page »

11) **Butt Kicks.** Lie on the stomach with the chin on the ground. Extend the arms straight forward on the ground, palms facing down. Alternately kick the buttocks with the heels in a steady rhythm as you chant **HAR** with each kick (2 kicks per second) for **1 minute**. (In the original class, Punjabi Drums were played to keep the rhythm.)

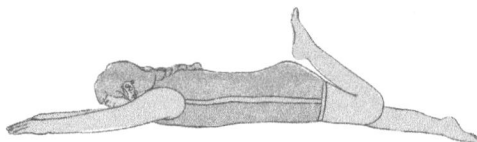

12) **Hit the Lower Back.** Remain on the stomach. Alternately hit the lower back with the hands in a steady rhythm as you chant **HAR** with each hit (1 hit per second) for **1 minute**. (In the original class, Punjabi Drums were played to keep the rhythm.)

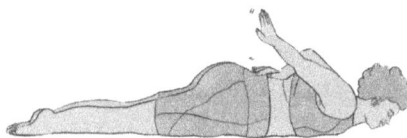

13) **Standing Side Bends.** Stand straight with the heels together and the feet open to 45 degrees. Interlace the fingers, raise the arms, and create an arc around the head. Bend from the waist to each side in a steady rhythm as you chant **HAR HARAY HAREE** (1 cycle and 1 repetition of the mantra per 2 seconds). Continue for **1 minute**. (In the original class, Punjabi Drums were played to keep the rhythm.)

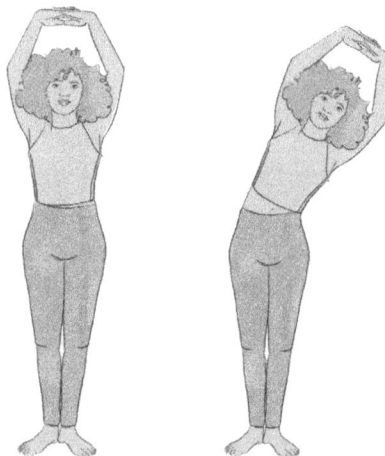

14) **Bowing Jaap Sahib.** Sit in Rock Pose with the knees spread wide, the spine straight, and a light Neck Lock. Rest the hands at the crease of the hips, with the fingers pointing inward and the elbows out to the sides. Sit still and listen to the introduction. When the first Pauri begins, bend at the hips as you bring the forehead to touch the ground. Bow down with the first word of each line and come back up on the second word. Pause in the up position during the breaks in the recitation. Continue for **4 ½ minutes**.

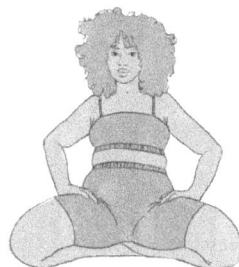

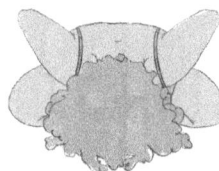

15) **Every Heartbeat Series.** a) Sit with the legs stretched forward and a straight spine. Bend from the hips, reach over the legs, and flex forward into Life Nerve Stretch. Grasp the big toes in a finger lock or hold where you can while maintaining an elongated spine and legs. Sing in the posture for **4 minutes**. (In the original class, the recording of "Every Heartbeat" by Nirinjan Kaur was played.)
b) Continue singing and move into Camel Pose. Come standing on your knees, hip-width apart. Lift the Heart Center and chest, bend back, and place the hands on the heels (or on the back of the thighs). Keep the pelvis over the knees and let the head

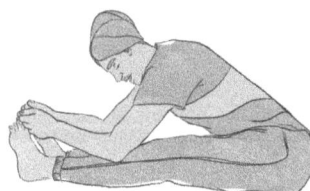

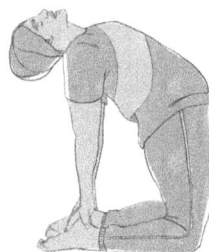

continue on next page »

drop back. Hold the position and sing for **1 ½ minutes**. c) Continue singing and move into Baby Pose. Sit on the knees and bend forward from the hips, placing the forehead on the ground with the arms along the sides, palms facing up. Continue to sing for **1 minute**. d) Stop singing and sleep in Baby Pose for **4 minutes**.

TO END: Inhale deeply as you come sitting up, then exhale. Repeat this breath **3 times**. Sit in Easy Pose, facing the sun. Relax the elbows by the sides, bring the forearms up, and angle the palms toward the sun. Close the eyes and let the sun shine on the eyelids and forehead. Continue for **30 seconds**. *Singing in the first posture of this series can make your voice very effective.*

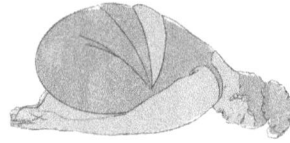

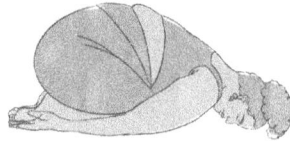

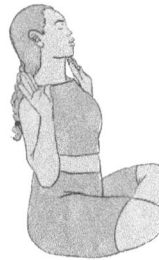

(14) Energizing Forward Flows

July 1, 1993

There are no breaks between exercises unless indicated.

1) **45-Degree Bend With Arm Circles.** Stand straight with the feet slightly wider than the shoulders and the feet open to a 45-degree angle. Bend forward from the hips to a 45-degree angle and stretch both arms out from the shoulder to the sides, palms facing down. Move the arms in 12-inch (31 cm) backward circles at a moderate pace. Continue for **3 minutes**. (In the original class, Punjabi Drums were played to keep the rhythm.) *Find balance in the upper body and the hips before beginning the arm movements. This exercise adjusts the ribcage, which brings harmony to the body and emotions.*

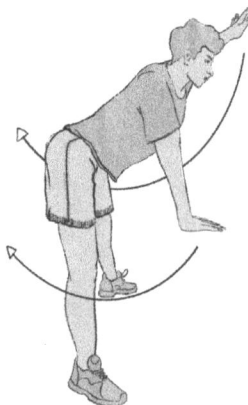

2) **Forward Bends With Arms at 45 Degrees.** Stand straight with the feet shoulder-width apart. Raise the right arm to a 45-degree angle, palm facing down. Bring the left arm back, palm facing up, creating a straight line with the arms. Bend forward from the hips, touch the ground with the right hand, and come back up. Maintain the straight line of the arms throughout the movement. Continue at a moderate pace (2 seconds per cycle) for **1 ½ minutes**. Switch sides and continue for **1 minute**.

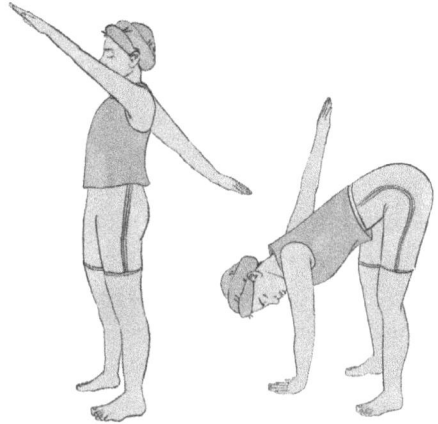

3) **Forward Bends Arms Open.** Stand straight with the feet slightly wider than the shoulders and bend forward from the hips to a 45-degree angle. Extend both arms open wide, parallel to the ground, palms facing down. Bend forward, touch the ground with both hands, and come back up. Keep the legs and spine straight. Move quickly (1 second per cycle) for **1 minute**.

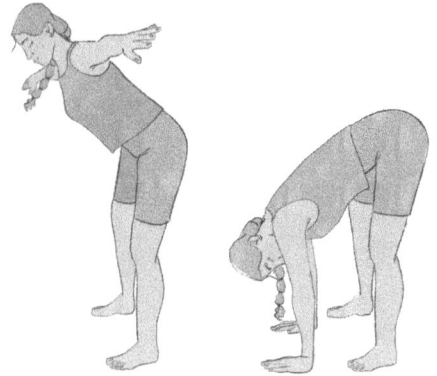

continue on next page »

4) **Jog In Place With Raised Fists.**
Stand straight and bend the elbows,
bringing the hands into fists by the
shoulders. Jog in place, raising the fist
straight up as you lift the opposite
knee high (the thigh is parallel to the
ground). Alternate legs and arms and
move at a fast pace for **2 minutes**.
Continue the movement and roar.
Let your anger out for **30 seconds**.
(In the original class, Punjabi Drums
were played to keep the rhythm.)

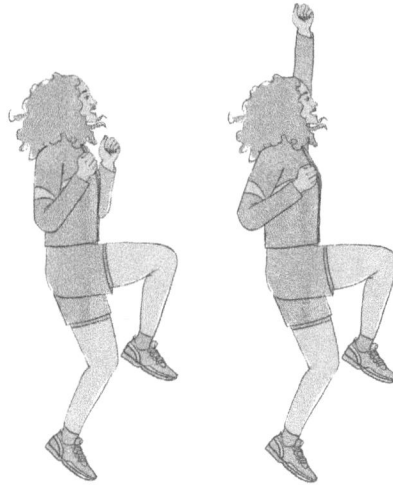

5) **Growling Lion.** Come onto hands
and knees, with palms on the ground
directly underneath the shoulders and
knees directly underneath the hips.
Open the mouth wide and stretch the
tongue out as far as it will go. Stare at
a point straight ahead and look like
an angry, attacking lion (If you have
a partner, stare into your partner's
eyes.) After **1 minute**, make a low
growling sound from the rib cage.
Continue for **1 ½ minutes**. Relax.
*When grief held in the rib cage is
lightened by physical exercise, you can
release anger and feel more relaxed.*

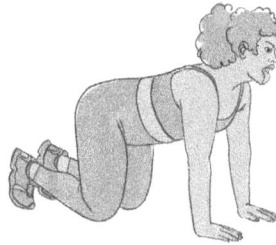

6) **Rock Forward and Back.** Sit in Rock Pose with the knees spread wide and the spine straight. Hold onto the elbows with the hands, locking them against the body. Close the eyes, rock forward to a 45-degree angle, and rock backward to a 45-degree angle. Move at a steady rhythm for **2 minutes**. Release the elbows and interlock the hands at the lower back. Continue the movement for **1 minute**. (In the original class, Punjabi Drums were played to keep the rhythm.)

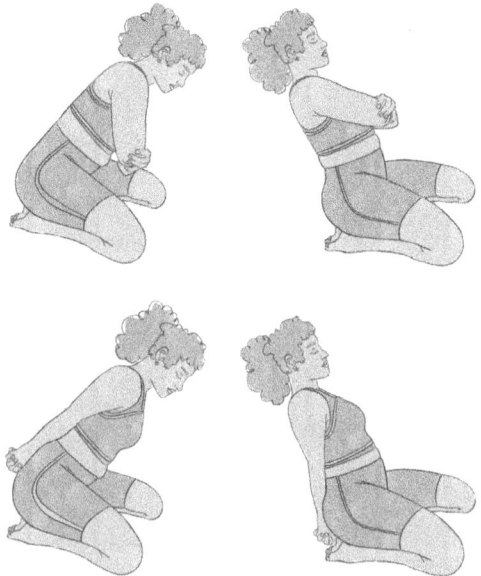

7) **Lotus Hands.** Remain in the posture and place the heels of the hands under the cheek bones. Open the fingers like a lotus flower; the fingers do not touch the head. Press and push up firmly. Keep the spine straight. Do not let the head bend backward with the pressure. Continue for **2 ½ minutes**.
You can massage the area with the heels of the palms while applying pressure.

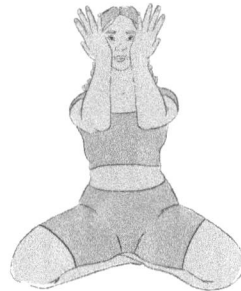

continue on next page »

8) **Arms Parallel Front and Back.**
Remain in the posture and extend
the left arm straight out in front of
the body, parallel to the ground,
palm facing down. Extend the right
arm straight back, parallel to the
ground, palm facing up. Hold the
posture for **1 ½ minutes**. Switch
sides and continue for **30 seconds**.
*When the arms are parallel to the
ground, sense that the energy flows
equally between the hands.*

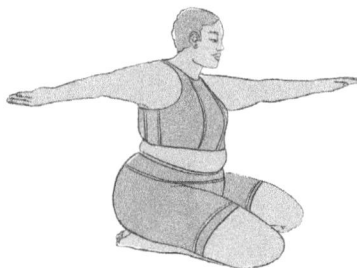

9) **Partner Wrestle.** ▲ Choose
a partner, and begin to wrestle.
Try to take the other person
down and pin them to the ground.
Continue for **1 ½ minutes**.

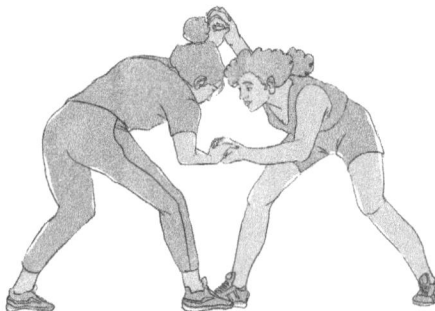

10) **Half Squat Meditation.** Stand
straight with the feet hip-width apart
and the toes open at a 45-degree
angle. Squat halfway down, with
the thighs parallel to the ground.
Support the body with the hands
on the knees, and keep the spine
straight and the head in line. Meditate
in this position for **3 ½ minutes**.
*Hypnotize yourself and conquer the
pain with the power of your brain.*

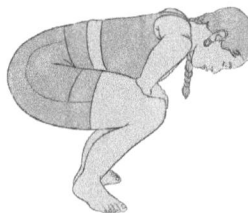

15 Half-Squat Workout for Strength and Flexibility

July 2, 1993

There are no breaks between exercises unless indicated.

1) **Half Squat Parallel Bend.** a) Stand with the feet slightly wider than the shoulders. Come into a half-squatting position, draw the knees towards each other, and lean forward from the waist so the spine is parallel to the ground. Interlace the fingers and hold the arms out in front of the body. Continue for **4 ½ minutes**. b) Stand up and relax for **30 seconds**, then return to the posture. Continue for **1 minute**. c) Stand up and hit the sides of the lower spine with the hands. Continue for **1 minute**. *This posture opens the sacral spine, which promotes health, energy, and optimal sleep.*

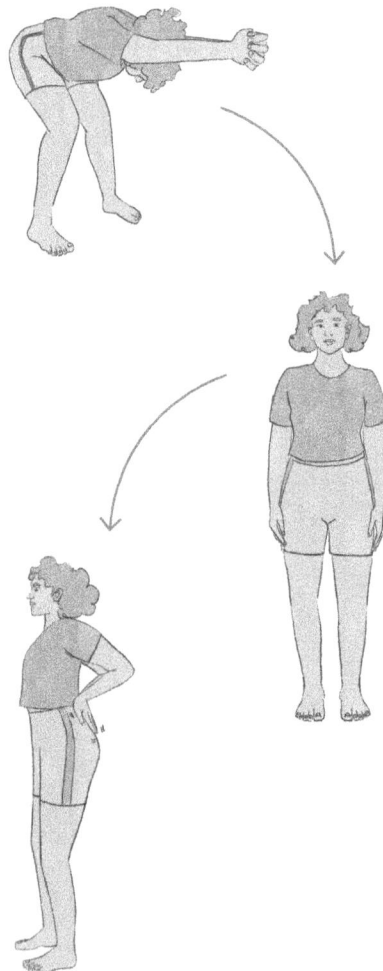

2) **Jumping Jacks.** Stand straight with the arms at your sides. Jump and open the legs wide as you bring both arms straight up and clap the hands over the head (1 clap per second). Jump again and bring the feet together and the arms down to your sides. Continue alternately jumping from one position to the other in a continuous motion for **1 ½ minutes**. (In the original class, Punjabi Drums were played to keep the rhythm.)

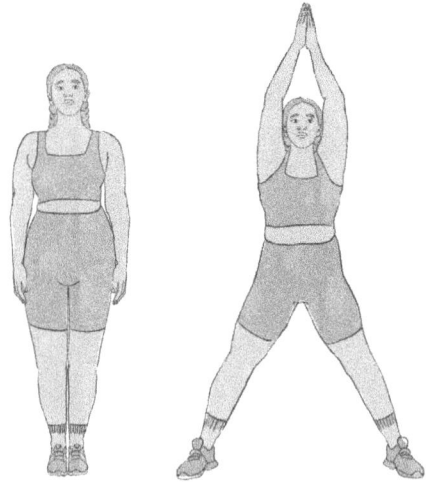

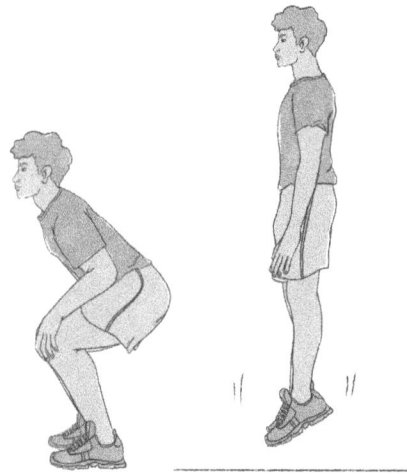

3) **Half Squat Jumps.** Come into a half squat, as in Exercise 1. Place the hands on the knees for support, and draw the knees towards each other. Straighten the legs, jump up, and return to the starting position. Continue for **1 ½ minutes**. (In the original class, Punjabi Drums were played to keep the rhythm.)

continue on next page »

4) **Triangle Pose Hips Side-to-Side.** Come into Triangle Pose with the feet wider than the hips. Place the hands on the ground in front of you, slightly wider than shoulder-width apart, approximately 30-36 inches (76-91 cm) from the feet. Keep the legs and arms straight. Move the hips rhythmically from side to side. Continue for **1 ½ minutes**. (In the original class, Punjabi Drums were played to keep the rhythm.)

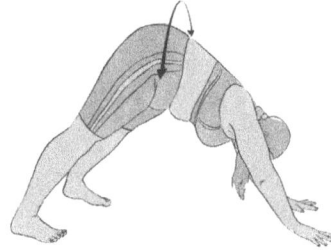

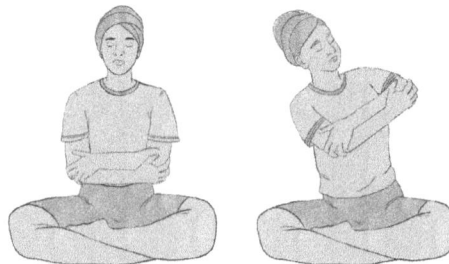

5) **Triangle Pose Dance.** Maintain the posture. Dance the hips to the music without lifting the hands or feet off the ground. Continue for **2 ½ minutes**. (In the original class, Punjabi Drums were played to keep the rhythm.) *This exercise develops the muscles in the lower spine to build stamina.*

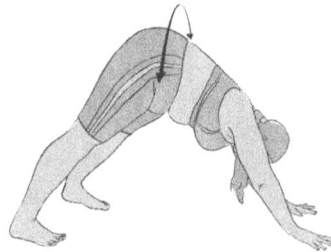

6) **Seated Dance.** Sit in Easy Pose with a straight spine. Hold onto opposite elbows, locking them in place. Close your eyes and dance the body wildly to the music without releasing the elbows. Continue for **3 minutes**. (In the original class, Punjabi Drums were played to keep the rhythm.)

7) **Frog Pose Dance.** Squat down in Frog Pose. Place the hands on the knees and dance to the music in this position. Continue for **1 ½ minutes**. (In the original class, Punjabi Drums were played to keep the rhythm.)

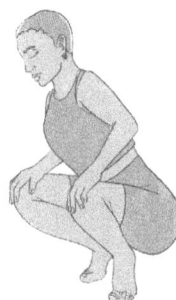

8) **Sit in the Sun.** Sit in Easy Pose with a straight spine and a light Neck Lock facing the sun. Relax the elbows by the sides, bring the forearms up, and angle the palms toward the sun. Close the eyes and let the sun shine on the eyelids and forehead. Chant the mantra **WHA-HAY GUROO, WHA-HAY GUROO, WHA-HAY GUROO, WHA-HAY JEEO**. Continue for **5 ½ minutes**. (In the original class, the recording by Wahe Guru Kaur was played.) *When practicing in a group, sit with no space in between people.*

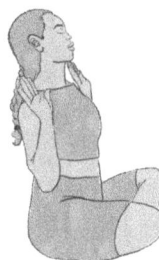

9) **Partner Wrestle. ▲** Choose a partner, and begin to wrestle. Try to take the other person down and pin them to the ground. Continue for **1 minute**.

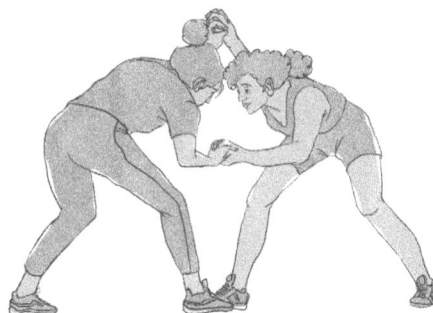

10) **Self-Hypnosis Meditation.**
a) Stand straight with the heels together. Bring the right hand beside the shoulder with the palm facing forward. Close the eyes. Stand still and reflect on your strength, dignity, nobility, passion, compassion, forgiveness, kindness, love, and friendship. Hypnotize yourself and mentally repeat the following words. Listen to your inner voice and believe yourself: **I AM IN LOVE, LOVE IN THE PURE FORM IS GREAT, I AM GREAT, I AM BEAUTIFUL, BOUNTIFUL, AND BLISSFUL.** Continue for **2 minutes**. b) Maintain the posture and sing with the music. Continue for **5 minutes**. (In the original class, "I Am Bountiful, Blissful and Beautiful" by Nirinjan Kaur from the Musical Affirmations Collection was played.)

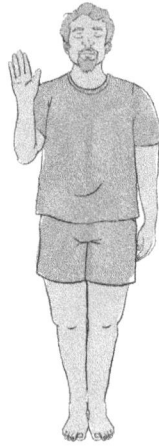

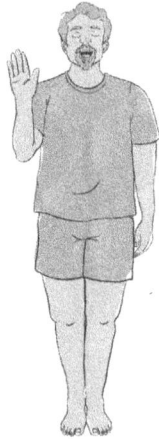

(16) Flowing Movement for Spinal Alignment

July 5, 1993

There are no breaks between exercises unless indicated.

1) **Alternate Arms and Butt Kicks.** Stand straight and raise the left arm up. Bend the right leg back to touch the buttocks. The right arm is relaxed at the side of the body. Balance in this posture for **1 minute**. Alternately raise arms and legs, kicking the buttocks with the heel in rhythm (1 second per movement). Continue the movement powerfully for **11 minutes**. (In the original class, Punjabi Drums were played to keep the rhythm.) Relax. *Kick the buttocks firmly and actively stretch the armpit with each repetition. The kick sets the hips; the arm movement balances the nervous system; and the chest and spine adjust automatically. This exercise keeps you physically, mentally, and spiritually balanced.*

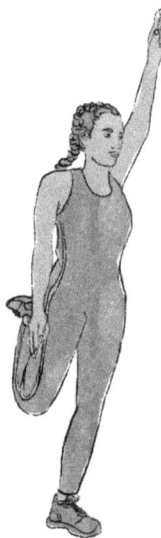

112

2) **Squat and Touch Ground.** Stand straight with the feet slightly wider than the hips and the feet open to a 45-degree angle. Squat down, touch the ground with both palms, and come back up. Keep the spine straight and the head in line. Continue at a pace of 2 seconds per cycle for **2 minutes**. (In the original class, Punjabi Drums were played to keep the rhythm.) *This exercise works on the first three vertebrae that relate to potential duality.*

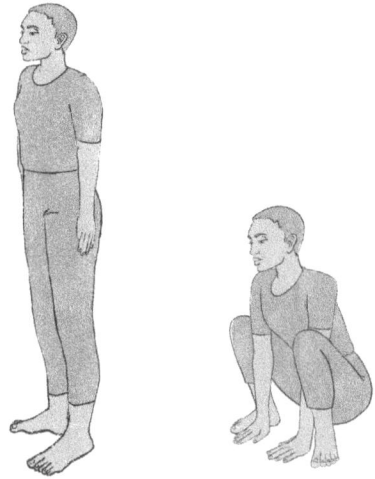

3) **Stand and Bend Back.** a) Stand straight with the heels touching and the feet open at a 45-degree angle. Interlock the hands behind the back. Lean back 60 degrees and come back upright. Keep the head in line with the body. Move in rhythm (2 seconds per cycle) for **1 minute**. b) Bend back, clap the hands in front of the body, then interlock them behind the back and come upright. Repeat this sequence (2 seconds per cycle) for **30 seconds**. (In the original class, Punjabi Drums were played to keep the rhythm.)

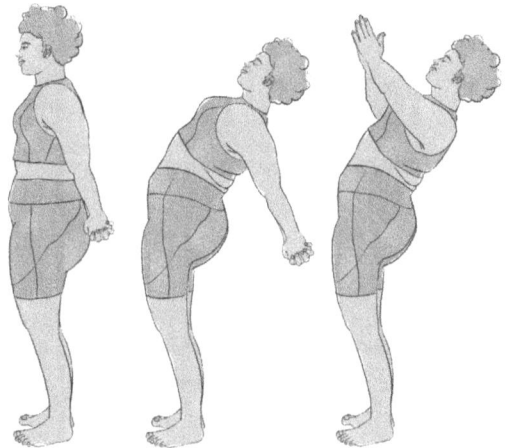

continue on next page »

4) **Pendulum Self-Hypnosis.** Sit in Rock Pose with the knees spread wide, the spine straight, and a light Neck Lock. Place the hands at the crease of the hips, with the fingers pointing inward and the elbows out to the sides. Close the eyes and imagine there is a pendulum in the frontal lobe of the brain. As the pendulum swings to one side, mentally repeat, 'I am not.' As the pendulum swings to the other side, mentally repeat, 'God is.' Hypnotize yourself and meditate for **5 ½ minutes**. (In the original class, "Say Saraswati" by Nirinjan Kaur was played.)

TO END: Inhale deeply, lean back 60 degrees, and suspend the breath for **30 seconds**. Mentally say a personal prayer. Exhale and relax. *This exercise works on the frontal lobe, the seat of personality in the brain, and stimulates the hammer bone of the inner ear, reinforcing self-hypnosis.*

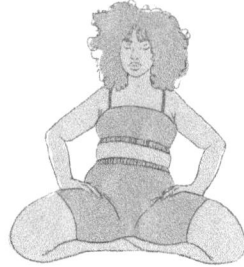

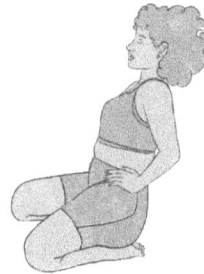

5) **Partner Wrestle.** ▲ Choose a partner, and begin to wrestle. Try to take the other person down and pin them to the ground. Continue for **30 seconds**.

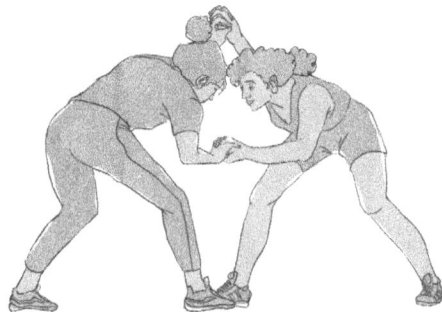

(17) Unleash Energy and Alignment

July 6, 1993

There are no breaks between exercises, unless indicated.

1) **Forward Bend With Arm Swings.**
Stand straight with the feet together.
Bend from the waist 40 degrees
forward. Make fists with both hands
and alternately swing the arms as
far forward and back as possible.
Keep the arms and legs straight and
the head in alignment with the body.
Move at a fast pace for **4 minutes**.
This exercise circulates the spinal fluid.

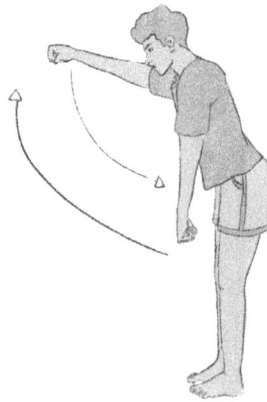

2) **Stand and Touch Ground.** Stand
straight with the heels together and
the feet open at a 45-degree angle.
Stretch the arms straight forward
with the palms facing down. Bend
forward from the hips and touch
the ground with both hands. Come
back up, keeping the legs and arms
straight and the head in alignment
with the body (2 seconds per cycle).
Breathe deeply with the movement.
Continue for **3 minutes**. Relax.

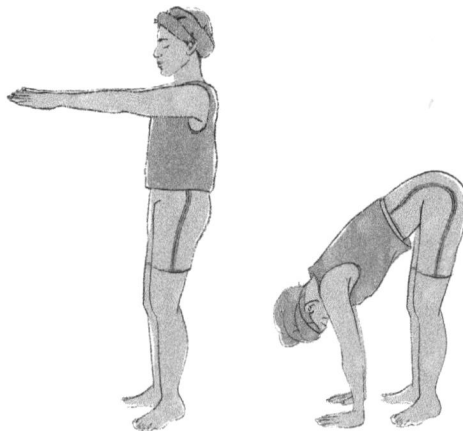

(In the original class, Punjabi Drums were played to keep the rhythm.) *The feet at 45 degrees stimulate liver and heart points.*

3) **Alternate Arms and Butt Kicks.** Stand straight. Raise the left arm up, palm facing forward, as you bend the right leg and kick the buttocks. Alternate arms and legs in rhythm (1 second per movement). Keep the arms straight and move powerfully. Continue for **3 ½ minutes**. (In the original class, Punjabi Drums were played to keep the rhythm.)

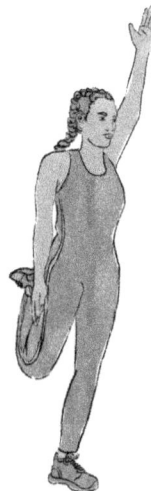

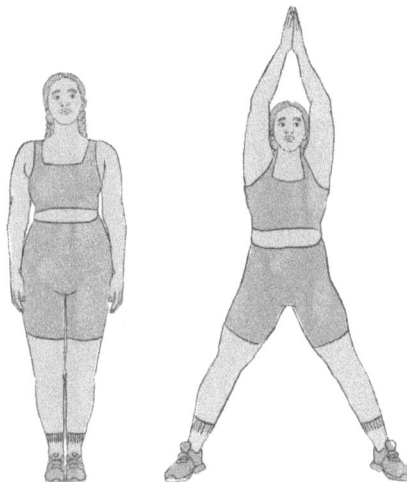

4) **Jumping Jacks.** Stand straight with the arms at your sides. Jump and open the legs wide as you bring both arms straight up and clap the hands over the head (1 clap per second). Jump again and bring the feet together and the arms down to your sides. Continue alternately jumping from one position to the other in a continuous motion for **3 minutes**. (In the original class, Punjabi Drums were played to keep the rhythm.)

continue on next page »

5) **Sit in the Sun With Sat Siree, Siree Akaal.** Sit in Easy Pose with a straight spine and a light Neck Lock facing the sun. Relax the elbows by the sides, bring the forearms up, and angle the palms toward the sun. Close the eyes and let the sun shine on the eyelids and forehead. Meditate and chant **SAT SIREE, SIREE AKAAL, SIREE AKAAL, MAAHAA AKAAL, MAAHAA AKAAL, SAT NAAM, AKAAL MOORAT, WHA-HAY GUROO**. Continue for **4 ½ minutes**. (In the original class, "Aquarian March" by Nirinjan Kaur from the White Tantra Yoga series was played.)

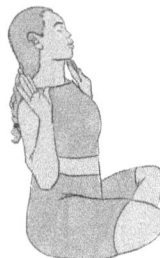

6) **Partner Wrestle.** ▲ Choose a partner, and begin to wrestle. Try to take the other person down and pin them to the ground. Continue for **1 minute**.

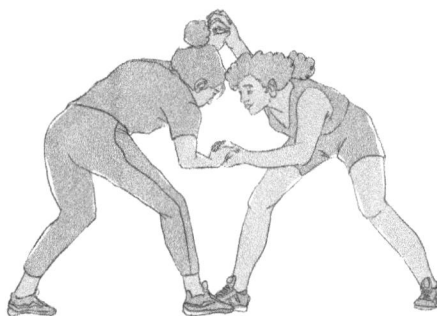

7) **Sit and Stand.** Stand up straight with the arms out straight forward, cross the ankles, and sit down in Easy Pose. Stand up again without using the hands for support. Alternate between standing and sitting (4 seconds per cycle) for **1 minute**.

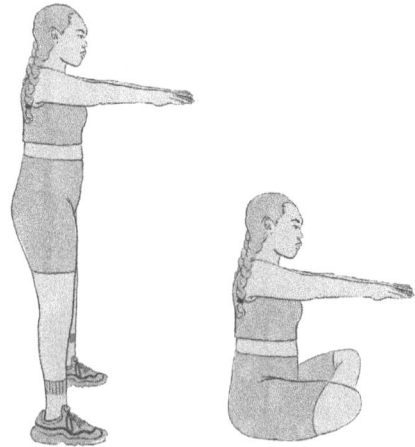

8) **Heart Meditation.** Sit in Rock Pose with the knees spread apart, a straight spine, and a light Neck Lock. Place both hands on the Heart Center, one on top of the other. Close the eyes and feel your strength. Realize your perfect self and perfect healing. Continue for **1 minute**.

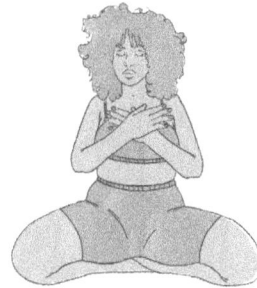

(18) Embrace Energy Through Movement

July 7, 1993

There are no pauses between exercises.

1) **One-Leg Balance.** Stand and raise your right leg back, keeping both legs straight. Bring the left arm straight forward and the right arm alongside the body. With all the weight on the left leg, lean forward and allow the body to balance, creating a straight line from the toes to the fingertips. Continue for **2 minutes**. Switch sides and hold the posture for **1 minute**.

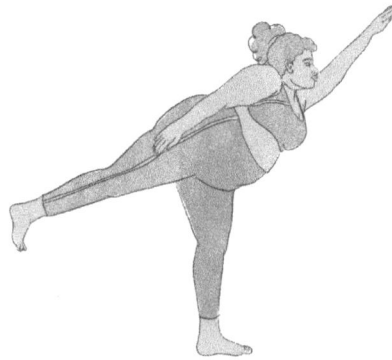

2) **Wide-Leg Half Squats.** Stand with the legs as wide apart as possible. Extend both arms straight forward, parallel to the ground, palms facing down. Bend the knees, squat down halfway, and come back up. Move in rhythm (one cycle per second) for **4 minutes**. (In the original class, Punjabi Drums were played to keep the rhythm.)

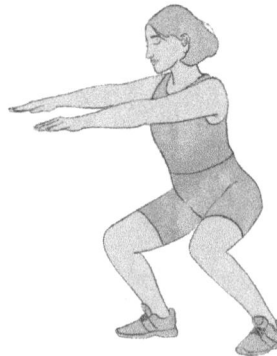

3) **Jog In Place.** Stand straight with the feet comfortably apart. Bend the elbows to 90 degrees, with the palms facing each other, held stiff and flat. Alternately move the arms forward and back from the shoulder as you jog in place, bringing the knees up high. Continue for **3 minutes**. (In the original class, Punjabi Drums were played to keep the rhythm.)

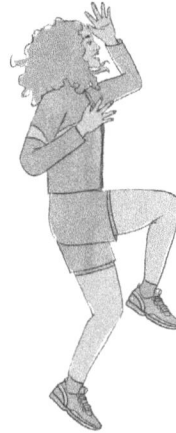

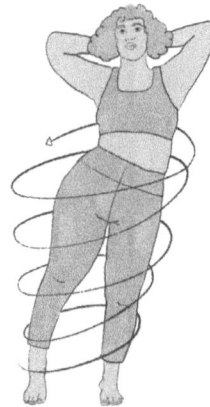

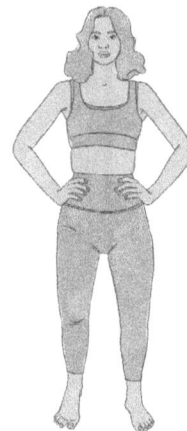

4) **Standing Body Circles.** Stand with the feet slightly wider than the shoulders. Interlace the fingers behind the neck with the elbows out to the sides. Rotate the lower body and legs from the ankles in clockwise circles. Continue for **2 minutes**. (In the original class, Punjabi Drums were played to keep the rhythm.)

5) **Step In Place.** Stand with the feet shoulder-width apart. Place the hands on the hips. Alternately lift one heel off the ground, shifting the weight to the opposite leg. Move quickly for **1 minute**. (In the original class, Punjabi Drums were played to keep the rhythm.)

continue on next page »

6) **Jumping Jacks.** Stand straight with the arms at your sides. Jump and open the legs wide as you bring both arms straight up and clap the hands over the head (1 clap per second). Jump again and bring the feet together and the arms down to your sides. Continue alternately jumping from one position to the other in a continuous motion for **2 ½ minutes**. (In the original class, Punjabi Drums were played to keep the rhythm.)

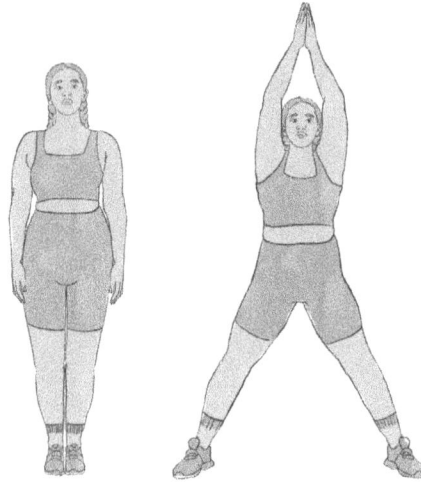

7) **Alternate Arms and Butt Kicks.** Stand straight. a) Raise the left arm up, palm facing forward, as you bend the right leg and kick the buttocks. Alternate arms and legs in rhythm (1 second per movement). Keep the arms straight and move powerfully. Continue for **1 minute**. b) Hold hands with your partner and continue the exercise. Lift the arms up in unison and kick the buttocks with the heels. Continue for **1 minute**. (In the original class, Punjabi Drums were played to keep the rhythm.) *If doing this exercise in a group, turn to stand facing a partner. (If you do not have a partner, continue the exercise solo.)*

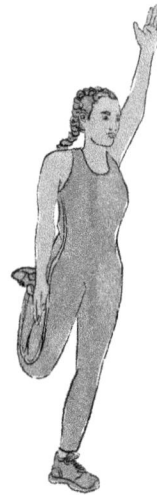

8) **Crow Squats.** Stand with the feet shoulder-width apart and the arms straight forward, palms facing down. Squat all the way down, then come back up. Keep the spine perpendicular to the ground. Continue for **2 minutes**. (In the original class, Punjabi Drums were played to keep the rhythm.) *If doing this exercise in a group, hold hands with your partner and squat down in unison.*

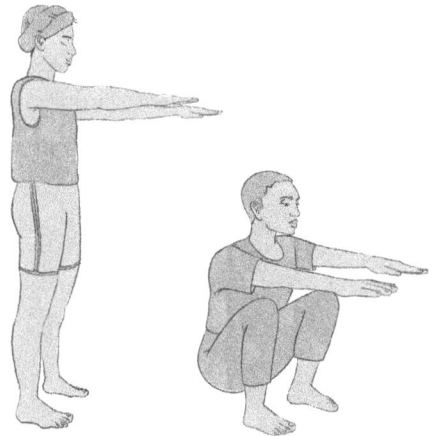

9) **Sing and Meditate.** Stand straight. a) Close the eyes and sing with the music. Continue for **5 ½ minutes**. b) Sit in Easy Pose with a straight spine and a light Neck Lock. Bring your hands into Prayer Pose. Keep the eyes closed and continue to sing with the music for **4 minutes**. (In the original class, "I Am Bountiful, Blissful and Beautiful" by Nirinjan Kaur from the Musical Affirmations Collection was played.) *If doing this exercise in a group, stand in a line and place your hands on the shoulders of the person on either side.*

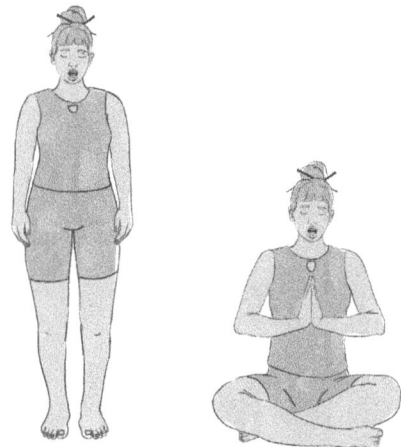

(19) Standing Bow Circuit for Graceful Alignment

July 8, 1993

There are no breaks between exercises, unless indicated.

1) **Sit and Stand.** Stand up straight with the arms straight forward, cross the ankles, and sit down in Easy Pose. Stand up again without using the hands for support. Alternate between standing and sitting. Continue (2 seconds per cycle) for **2 ½ minutes**. Place both hands on the Heart Center, and continue for **11 repetitions**. Relax.

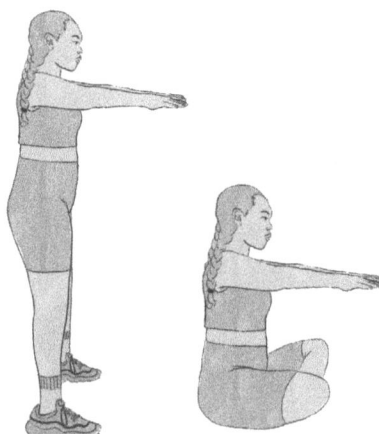

2) **Side-to-Side Rolls.** Lie on the stomach with the arms by the sides. Roll on the torso and legs from left to right without rolling onto the back. Continue (2 seconds per cycle) for **4 minutes**. (In the original class, Punjabi Drums were played to keep the rhythm.)
This exercise adjusts the skeletal system.

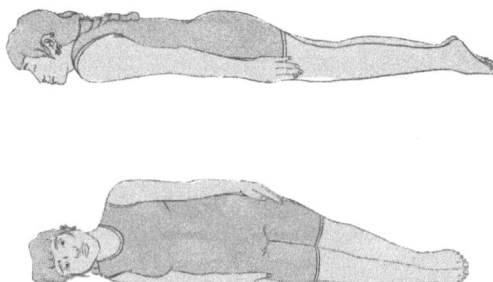

3) **Sitting Jumps.** a) Sit in Easy Pose and jump up and down without using the hands. Lift the buttocks off the ground in rhythm (2-3 jumps per second). Continue for **2 ½ minutes**. b) Come onto the heels in Rock Pose with the knees spread wide. Place the hands on the shoulders with the fingers in front and the thumbs in back, elbows out to the sides. Strongly pull the navel in and jump up, rhythmically lifting the buttocks up and down on the heels (2-3 jumps per second). Continue for **3 ½ minutes**. (In the original class, Punjabi Drums were played to keep the rhythm.) Relax. *This movement works the Navel Point and awakens the Kundalini energy.*

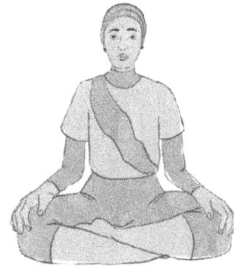

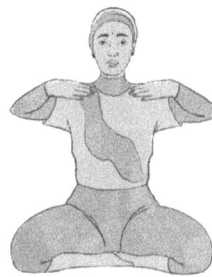

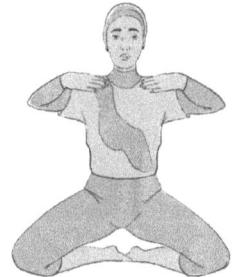

4) **Rise Up in Rock Pose.** a) Remain in the Rock Pose and interlace the fingers together behind the neck. Rise up to standing on the knees and come sitting back down. Move in rhythm (1 cycle per 2 seconds). Continue for **2 minutes**. b) Remain in the posture and interlock the hands overhead. Continue for **1 minute**. (In the original class, Punjabi Drums were played to keep the rhythm.)

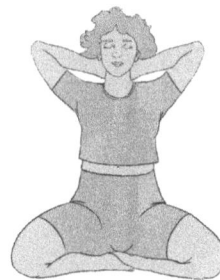

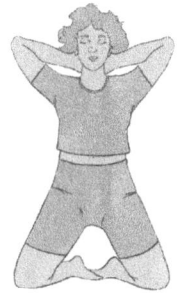

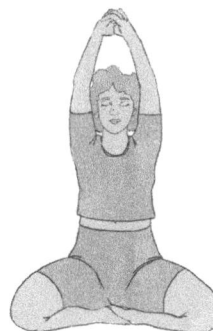

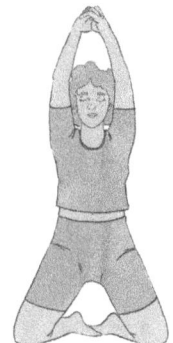

continue on next page »

5) **Bow in Rhythm.** Remain in the posture with the arms straight overhead, with palms facing forward. Bend forward, touch the palms and forehead to the ground, and come back up. Keep the arms in alignment with the body. Move at a steady pace in rhythm (2 seconds per cycle). Continue for **1 minute**. (In the original class, Punjabi Drums were played to keep the rhythm.) *As you move, you can use the affirmation "I bow (bowing down), ego (coming up)."*

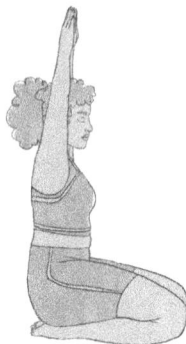

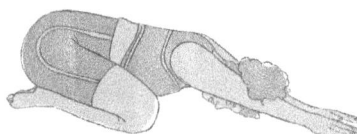

6) **Sit in the Sun.** Sit in Easy Pose with a straight spine and a light Neck Lock facing the sun. Relax the elbows by the sides, bring the forearms up, and angle the palms toward the sun. Close the eyes and let the sun shine on the eyelids and forehead. Create a self-hypnosis that you are beautiful, bountiful, and blissful. Continue for **7 minutes**. (In the original class, "I Am Bountiful, Blissful and Beautiful' by Nirinjan Kaur from the Musical Affirmations Collection was played.) Relax.

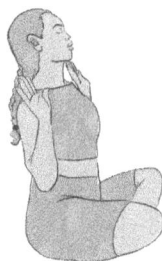

7) **Partner Wrestle.** ▲ Choose a partner, and begin to wrestle. Try to take the other person down and pin them to the ground. Continue for **1 minute**.

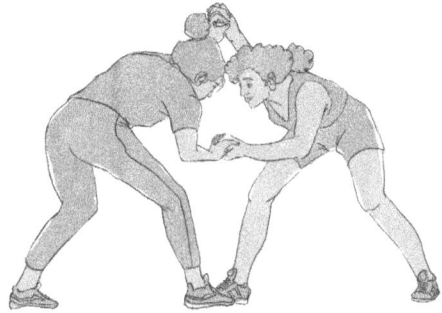

8) **Standing Bow.** Stand straight with the heels together and the feet open at a 45-degree angle, arms at the sides. Bow forward, bringing the back parallel to the ground. Hold this position for **2 seconds**, and come back up. The arms remain at the sides throughout. Continue for **11 repetitions**.

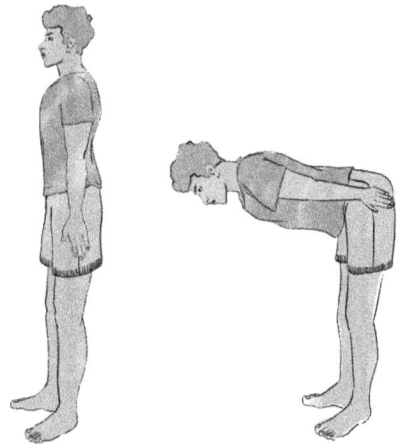

(20) Bends and Swings for Vitality

July 9, 1993

There are no pauses between exercises.

1) **Forward Bend With Arm Swings.** a) Stand straight with the heels together and the feet open at a 45-degree angle, arms at the sides. Bend forward from the hips to a 60-degree angle. Keep the spine straight and the head in alignment with the body. Hold for **2 ½ minutes**. b) Swing the arms alternately forward and backward. Keep the arms straight and move fast for **4 minutes**.
This exercise works on the shoulders and the neck and can prevent headaches.

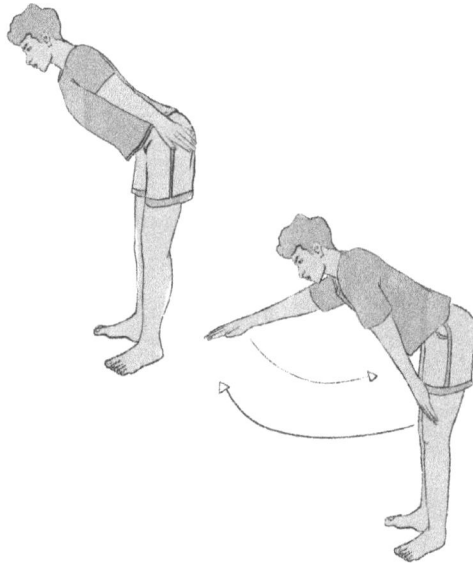

2) **Backward Bend With Arm Swings.** Remain standing and bend backward to a 40-degree angle. Begin to swing the arms alternately forward and backward. Keep the arms straight and move fast for **1 ½ minutes**.
This exercise opens circulation to the chest area.

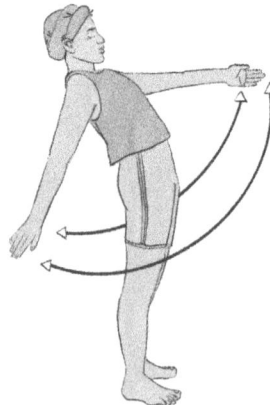

3) **Sit and Stand.** Stand up straight with the arms straight forward, cross the ankles, and sit down in Easy Pose. Stand up again without using the hands for support. Alternate between standing and sitting for **6 minutes**. *If doing this exercise in a class setting, the teacher instructs the students to sit and stand at random intervals. This trains the physical body to respond quickly.*

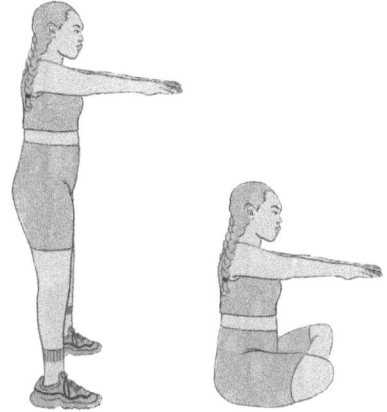

4) **Shuniya Meditation.** Sit in Easy Pose with a straight spine and a light Neck Lock. Hold onto the knees and lean backward to a 40-degree angle. Close the eyes and consciously release any angry, fearful, or unbalanced thoughts; drop emotional baggage. Bring everything to oneness, or Shuniya. Meditate for **5 ½ minutes**.

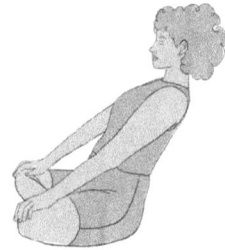

5) **Jumping Jacks.** Stand straight with the arms at your sides. Jump and open the legs wide as you bring both arms straight up and clap the hands over the head (1 clap per second). Jump again and bring the feet together and the arms down to your sides. Continue alternately jumping from one position to the other in a continuous motion for **9 ½ minutes**. (In the original class, Punjabi Drums were played to keep the rhythm.)

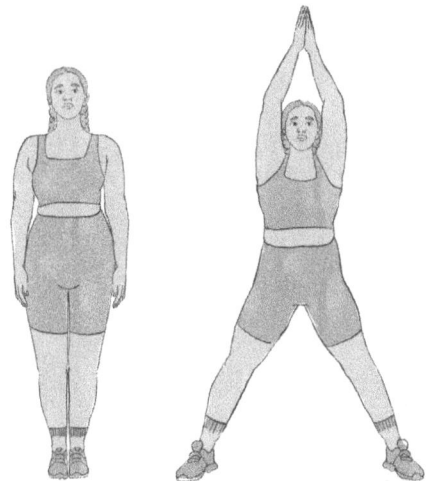

continue on next page »

6) **Aquarian Mantra Meditation.** Sit in Rock Pose with the knees spread wide, the spine straight, and a light Neck Lock. Place the hands at the crease of the hips, with the fingers pointing inward and the elbows out to the sides. Close the eyes, meditate and chant the Aquarian Sadhana mantras[6] from **WAAH YANTEE** through **WHAA-HAY GUROO WHAA-HAY JEEO** for **40 minutes.** (In the original class, Aquarian Sadhana mantras by Seva Kaur were played.)

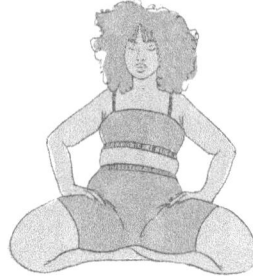

7) **Relaxation.** Lie on the stomach with the arms by the sides. Relax and sleep in this posture for **3 minutes**. (In the original class, the recording "Wahe Guru Wahe Jeeo" by Seva Kaur was played.)

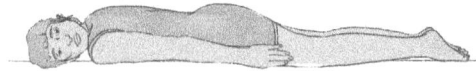

6   You can find all Aquarian Sadhana mantras in the appendix, on page 226.

(21) Twist, Bow and Squat Workout

June 27, 1994

There are no breaks between exercises, unless indicated.

1) **Squats With Heels Together.** Stand straight with the heels together and the feet open at a 45-degree angle. Interlace the fingers behind the head at the hairline under any loose hair, elbows stretched out to the sides. Squat all the way down, then come back up. Keep the spine perpendicular to the ground. Continue for **2 minutes**.

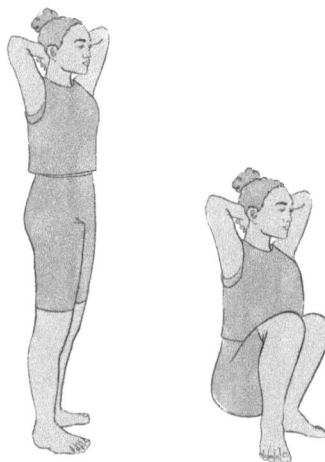

2) **Squat & Bow Series.** Remain standing with the hands behind the neck. Begin a 6-part series: a) Squat down; b) Lie on the stomach with the arms stretched forward on the ground, palms facing down; c) Grasp the ankles and lift up into Bow Pose; d) Lie on the stomach as before; e) Squat; and f) Come standing up. Continue this series for **2 minutes**.

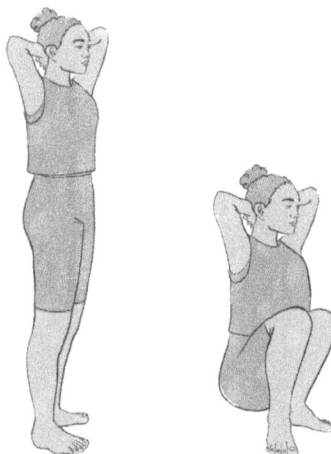

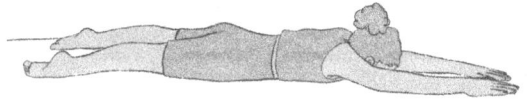

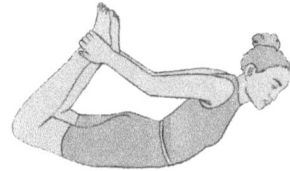

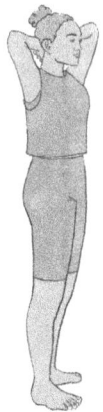

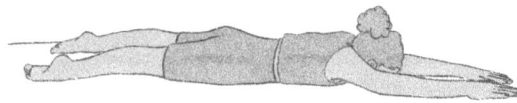

3) **Rocking Bow & Squat Series.**
a) Rock back and forth on the stomach in Bow Pose for **1 ½ minutes**. End by lying flat on the stomach, squatting, and then standing up. b) Squat down and stand up alternately for **30 seconds**. c) Lie on the stomach with the arms stretched forward on the ground, grasp the ankles, and lift up into Bow Pose. Rock back and forth on the stomach for **30 seconds**.

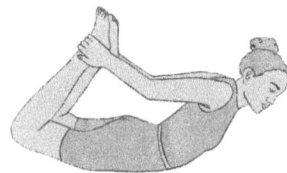

continue on next page »

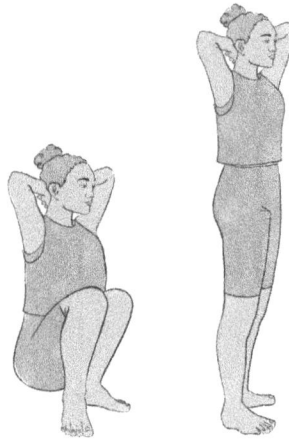

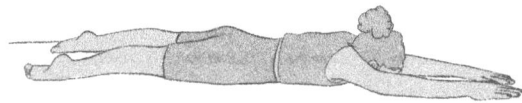

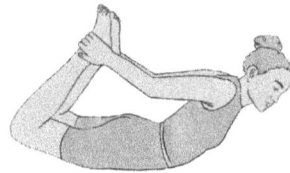

4) **Standing Torso Twist.** Stand with the hands interlaced behind the neck. Twist the body from side to side rapidly (1 second per cycle) for **1 minute**.

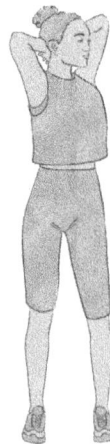

5) **Stand and Touch Ground.** Stand straight with the heels together and the feet open at a 45-degree angle. Stretch the arms straight forward with the palms facing down. Bend forward from the hips and touch the ground with both hands. Come back up, keeping the legs and arms straight and the head in alignment with the body (2 seconds per cycle). Breathe deeply with the movement. Continue for **1 ½ minutes**. *In the first few repetitions, pause, touching the ground, and stretch the tailbone.*

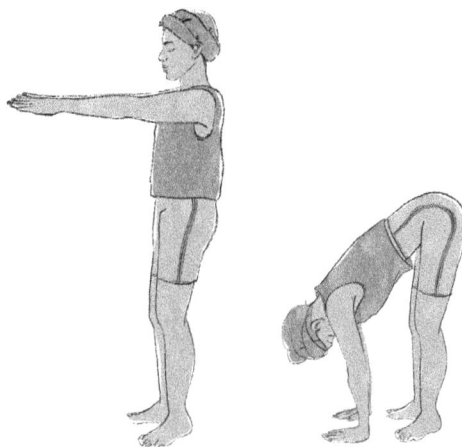

6) **Elephant Walk.** Stand straight and fold forward from the hips to touch the ground with both hands. Walk around on all fours, keeping the legs straight. Continue for **2 minutes**. *If practicing alone, talk to yourself. If doing this exercise in a group, greet and talk to each other as you walk around.*

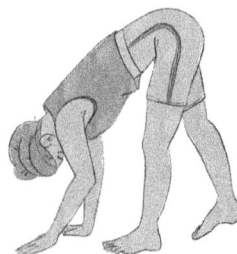

7) **Sing in Corpse Pose.** a) Relax on the back in Corpse Pose with arms at the sides and palms facing up for **1 minute**. b) Sing the national anthem of your country for **2 ½ minutes**.

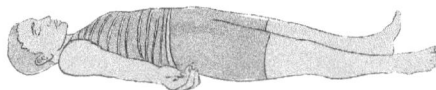

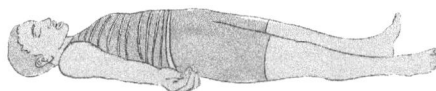

continue on next page »

8) **Wide Leg Hold.** Remain on the back, bring the legs up to 90 degrees, and open them into a wide V shape. Hold for **1 minute**.
TO END: Bring the legs together, lift the weight onto the shoulders, and bring the feet overhead towards the ground behind you, coming into Plow Pose. Keep the legs together and straight. Hold for **30 seconds**. *This posture adjusts the lower back and helps prevent disease.*

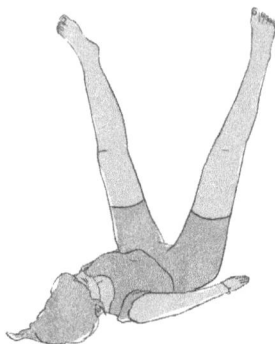

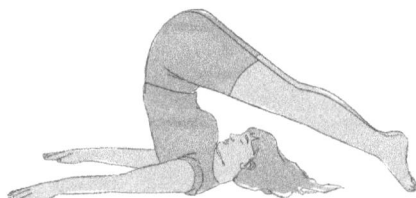

9) **Sing in Baby Pose.** Sit on the heels in Rock Pose and bend forward, placing the forehead on the ground and relaxing the shoulders. The arms are by the sides, palms facing up. Sing the national anthem of your country in this posture for **1 ½ minutes**.

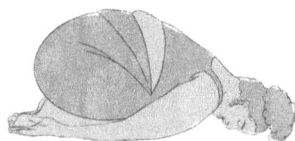

(22) Release Negative Thoughts, Rejoice and Relax

June 28, 1994

There are no pauses between exercises.

1) **Parallel Forward Bend Series.** Stand straight with the feet a little wider than shoulder width. Stretch the arms straight up, palms facing forward. a) Slowly bend from the hips until the torso and arms are parallel to the ground. Actively stretch forward with the arms and head and backward with the hips; create a balance. Keep the arms, legs, and spine straight; tilt the head up to look forward. Continue for **3 minutes**. b) Maintaining the arm position, come up straight and stretch up and back. Hold the stretch for **30 seconds**. c) Bend forward from the hips as in posture (a) and hold for **30 seconds**. d) Maintaining the arm position, come up straight and stretch up and back as in posture (b). Hold the stretch for **30 seconds**. e) Bend forward from the hips as in posture (a). f) Keeping the torso and arms

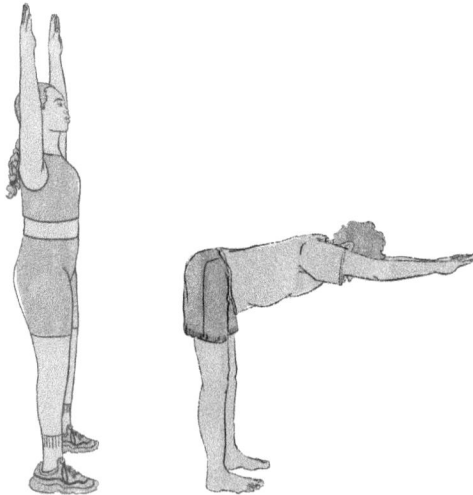

parallel to the ground, move from the Parallel Forward Bend position into a squat, then return to the starting position. Continue alternating between postures (e) and (f) for **1 minute**. *This exercise can unlock the pelvic diaphragm and help prevent lower back pain.*

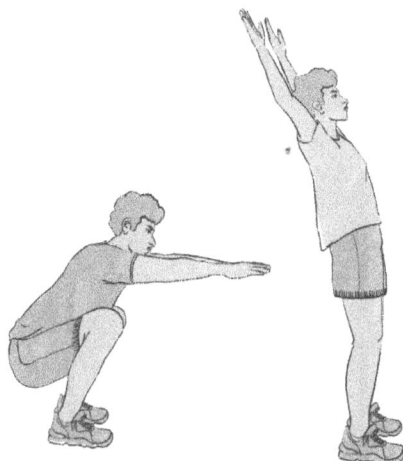

2) **Bow Pose.** Lie on the stomach, keeping the knees in line with or slightly wider than the hips. Reach back and grasp the ankles. With the arms straight, lengthen the spine and lift the Heart Center, head, and thighs off the ground. Press down through the pelvis, use the legs to pull, and stretch up into Bow Pose with a long neck. Rock back and forth from shoulder to hip. Make up a song about all the negative things in life and sing it. Yell, scream, and cry; let out all the pain and sorrow. Continue for **3 minutes**.

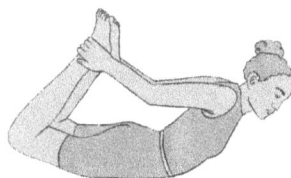

3) **Crying.** Sit in Easy Pose. Cover the face with the hands and cry loudly. Get it out for **1 minute**.

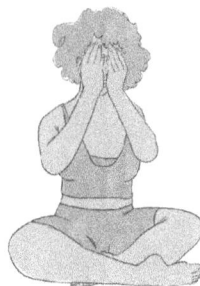

continue on next page »

4) **Laughing.** Remain in Easy Pose and relax the hands down. Tilt the face upward and laugh out loud. Continue for **30 seconds**.

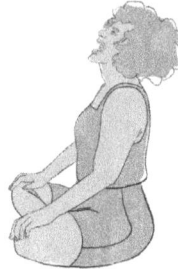

5) **Shoulder Stand Series.** a) Lie on the back. Bend the knees in toward the chest, shift the weight onto the shoulders, and lift the legs up straight to come into Shoulder Stand. Place the elbows on the ground, and use the hands to support the back. Cycle the legs in this posture for **1 minute**. b) Remain in the posture and alternately kick the buttocks with the heels. Continue to kick and sing the national anthem of your country for **2 ½ minutes**.

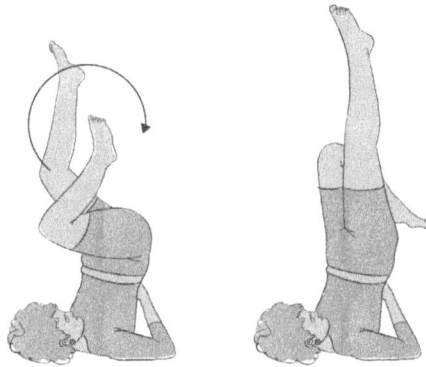

6) **Eyes Closed Walk.** Stand up, close the eyes, and hold the hands out in front. Walk around with the eyes closed for **2 minutes**. *If doing this exercise in a group, introduce yourself to everyone you encounter, keeping the eyes closed. Say hello, give your name, and then move on quickly.*

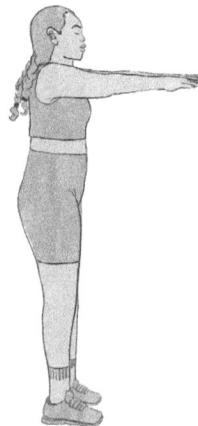

7) **Bhangra Dance.** Stand up and dance to the music. Keep the arms raised above the Heart Center, move the shoulders up and down, and shift the weight from one foot to the other so that one foot is always off the ground. Continue for **4 minutes**. (In the original class, Bhangra music was played.)

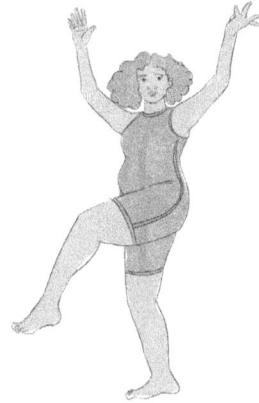

8) **Sit in the Sun.** Sit in Easy Pose with a straight spine and a light Neck Lock facing the sun. Relax the elbows by the sides, bring the forearms up, and angle the palms toward the sun. Close the eyes and let the sun shine on the eyelids and forehead. Meditate and chant **ONG NAMO GUROO DAYV NAMO**. Continue for **2 minutes**. (In the original class, the recording "Ong Namo Guru Dev Namo" by Nirinjan Kaur from the Tantric Meditation Series was played.)

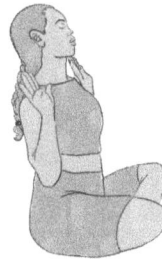

(23) Invigorating Balance and Strength Flow

June 29, 1994

There are no pauses between exercises.

1) **Archer Pose Stretch.** Stand and bring one leg forward with the knee bent at 90 degrees; the other leg remains straight. Bring the palms together in front of the body with the arms parallel to the ground. Hold the posture for **5 seconds**, then switch sides. Continue alternating sides for **1 ½ minutes**.

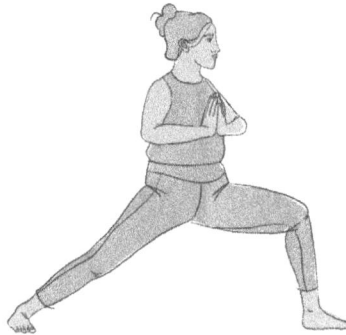

2) **Wide Leg Forward Bend Series.** a) Stand with the feet one yard apart (around 90 cm) and the hands on the hips. Bend forward from the hips as far as possible, then come back up to the starting position. Continue (one cycle per 2 seconds) for **1 minute**. b) Spread the feet even wider apart, point the toes outward, and continue for **30 seconds**. c) Interlace the hands behind the neck and continue for **30 seconds**. d) Stretch the hands straight forward from the shoulders and continue for **15 seconds**.

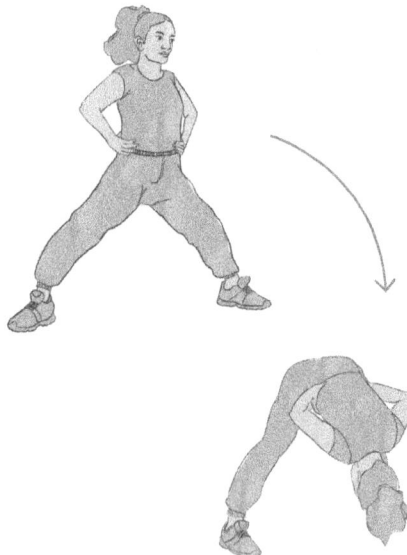

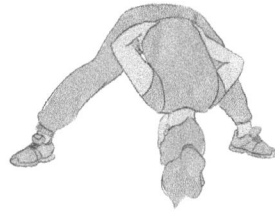

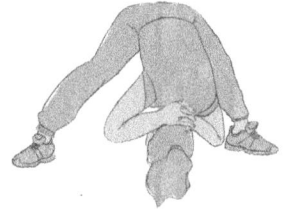

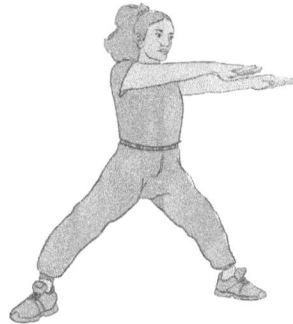

3) **Walk on All Fours.** Remain standing with feet wide apart, bend forward from the hips, and place both hands flat on the ground. Walk in place on all fours, keeping the legs and arms straight. Move from the hips for **4 minutes**. (In the original class, Punjabi Drums were played to keep the rhythm.)

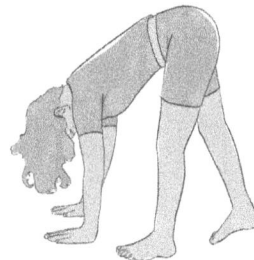

continue on next page »

4) **Hop on Alternate Feet.** Stand straight and hop from side to side, from one foot to the other. Swing the arms forward and back or up and down in rhythm with the movement for **9 minutes**. (In the original class, Punjabi Drums were played to keep the rhythm.) *If doing this exercise in a group setting, hold hands and hop with a partner for the last minute.*

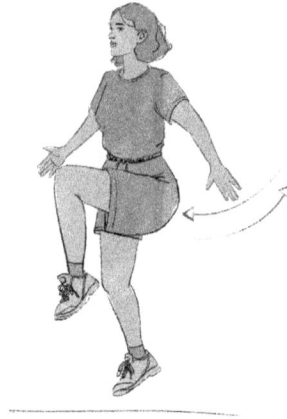

5) **Crossed Leg Lifts.** a) Lie on the back and cross the legs at the ankle. Raise both legs, with the ankles still crossed, up to 90 degrees, then separate the legs wide and cross them the opposite way. Lower the crossed legs down. Continue this series for **30 seconds**. b) Raise both legs, with the ankles still crossed, up to 90 degrees, then lower them again. Cross them the opposite way, then raise and lower them with the ankles still crossed. Continue this series for **30 seconds**.

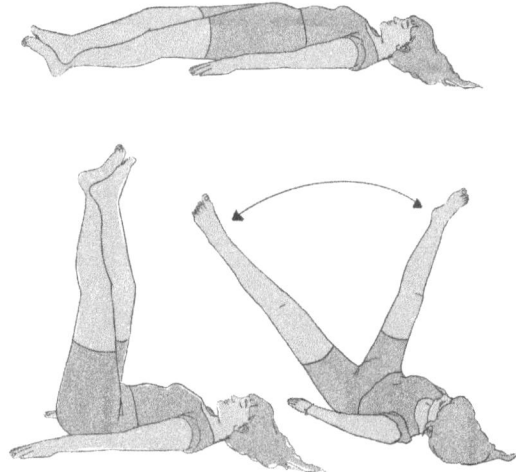

6) **Bow Pose Jumps.** Lie on the stomach, bend the knees, and reach back to grasp the ankles. Stretch up into Bow Pose and jump up and down in the posture. Continue for **1 minute**.

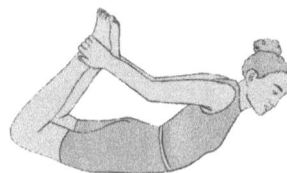

7) **Butt Kicks.** Lie on the back, lift the knees up, and alternately kick the buttocks with the heels. Continue for **1 minute**.

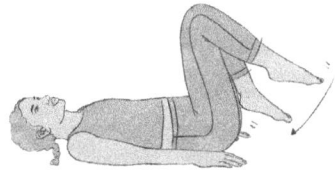

8) **Bicycle Arms and Legs.** Remain in the posture and move the arms and legs alternately in circles. Move fast and powerfully for **1 minute**.

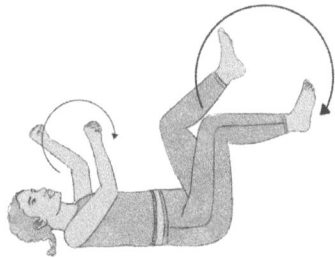

9) **Partner Wrestle.** ▲ Choose a partner, and begin to wrestle. Try to take the other person down and pin them to the ground. Continue for **1 minute**.

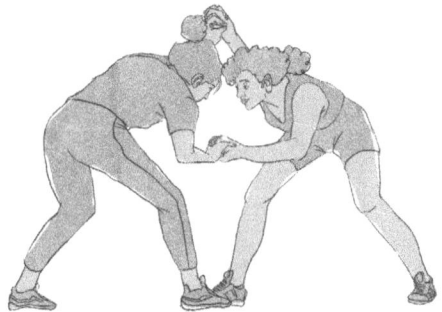

continue on next page »

10) **Clap Series.** Sit facing a partner and look into each other's eyes. a) Clap your hands together in front of the chest. b) Clap hands with your partner. c) Clap your hands together up high. d) Clap your partner's hands. Continue this 4 part sequence for **1 minute**. *If doing the exercise by yourself, clap against a wall or the ground instead of a partner's hands.*

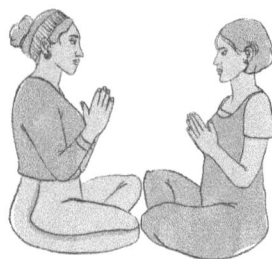

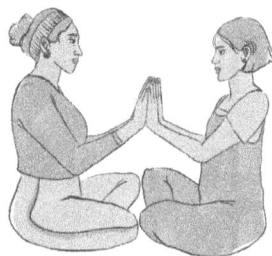

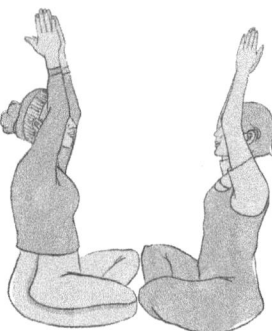

11) **Partner Wrestle. ▲** Stand up, choose a partner and firmly hold their shoulders. Push, pull, and move your partner around without losing the grip on the shoulders for **2 minutes.**

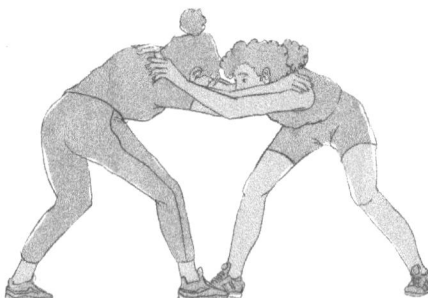

12) **Sit and Stand.** Stand straight and raise the arms straight overhead.
a) Sit down in Easy Pose. Stand up again without using the hands for support. Alternate between standing and sitting for **2 ½ minutes**.
b) Interlock hands with a partner and sit and stand in unison for **30 seconds**.

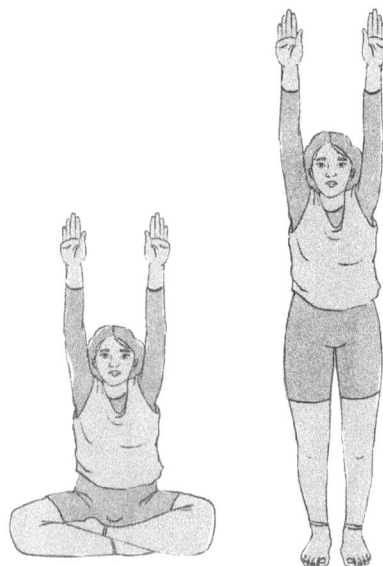

13) **Bhangra Dance.** Stand up and dance to the music. Keep the arms raised above the Heart Center, move the shoulders up and down, and shift the weight from one foot to the other so that one foot is always off the ground. Continue for **2 minutes**. (In the original class, Bhangra music was played.

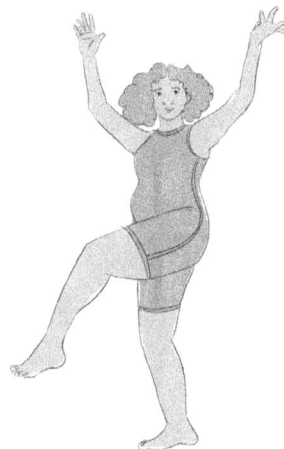

14) **Sit in the Sun.** Sit in Easy Pose with a straight spine and a light Neck Lock facing the sun. Relax the elbows by the sides, bring the forearms up, and angle the palms toward the sun. Close the eyes and let the sun

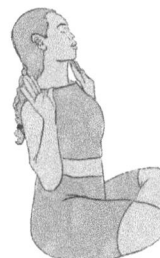

continue on next page »

shine on the eyelids and forehead. Meditate and chant **ONG NAMO GUROO DAYV NAMO**. Continue for **8 minutes**. (In the original class, the recording "Ong Namo Guru Dev Namo" by Nirinjan Kaur from the Tantric Meditation Series was played.) TO END: Inhale deeply and suspend the breath. Canon Fire exhale.

15) **Breath of Fire.** Remain seated. Breathe rapidly, rhythmically, and strongly through the nose. The breath is equal on the inhale and the exhale, with no pause between them. With each inhale, allow the navel to move naturally inward and upward. Release the navel on the exhale. Continue for **1 minute**.

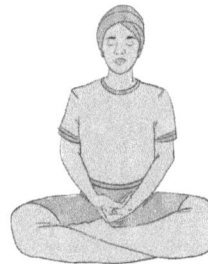

(24) Bounce and Balance for Relaxation and Strength

June 30, 1994

There are no pauses between exercises, except when indicated otherwise.

1) **Forward Bend With Arm Swings.** Stand with the feet shoulder-width apart. Bend forward, with the upper body parallel to the ground and the arms hanging down. Keep the legs and spine straight and look forward. Swing both arms together in an arc from left to right. Move powerfully so that the body twists with the movement. Continue for **4 minutes**.

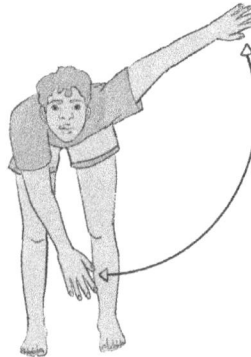

2) **Self-Wrestle.** ▲ Sit in Easy Pose and wrestle with yourself, try to bring yourself to the ground. Use your arms and legs to struggle against yourself. Continue for **3 minutes**. *This exercise relaxes you.*

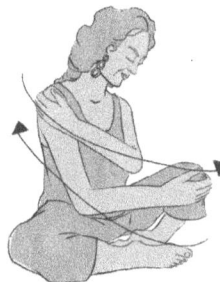

3) **Jump on All Fours.** Stand on your hands and feet with equal weight. Jump up and down so all four leave and return to the ground at the same time. Continue for **2 minutes**.

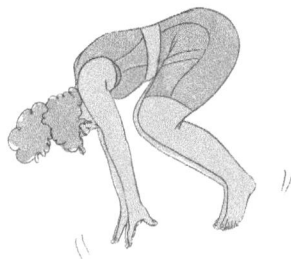

4) **Bhangra Dance.** Stand up and dance to the music. Keep the arms raised above the head, and move the shoulders up and down. Move the body in rhythm with the music and shift the weight from one foot to the other so that one foot is always off the ground. Continue for **3 minutes**. Relax. (In the original class, bhangra music was played.)

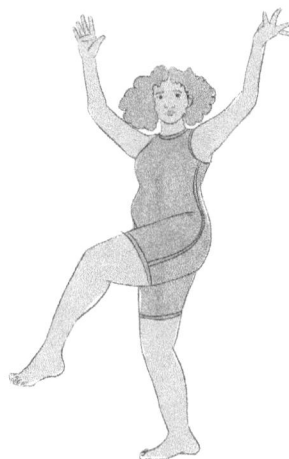

5) **Mesmerize.** Sit face-to-face in Easy Pose with a partner. Bring the hands forward until your palms meet your partner's. Look straight into your partner's eyes. Project psychically to the other person. Continue for **11 minutes**. (In the original class, Punjabi Drums were played to keep the rhythm.)
If practicing alone, imagine that you're mesmerizing a partner.

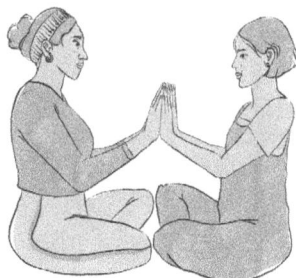

continue on next page »

6) **Partner Wrestle.** ▲ Choose a partner, and begin to wrestle. Try to take the other person down and pin them to the ground. Continue for **1 minute**. Relax.

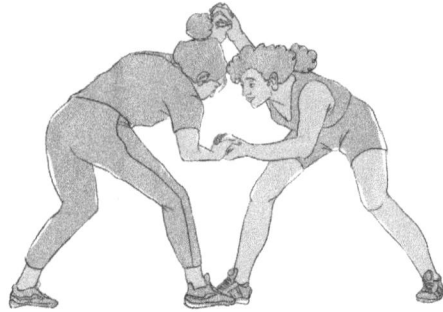

7) **Sit in the Sun.** Sit in Easy Pose with a straight spine and a light Neck Lock facing the sun. Relax the elbows by the sides, bring the forearms up, and angle the palms toward the sun. Close the eyes and let the sun shine on the eyelids and forehead. Chant **GURDAYV MAATAA GURDAYV PITAA**[7] from the heart for **11 minutes**.

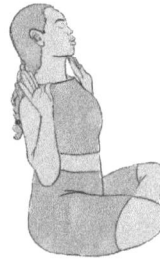

7   This mantra translates as "Divine Guru is my mother, Divine Guru is my father; Divine Guru is my transcendent Lord and Master. Divine Guru is my companion, the destroyer of ignorance; Divine Guru is my relative and brother. Divine Guru is the Giver, the Teacher of the Lord's Name. Divine Guru is the mantra that never fails. Divine guru is the image of peace, truth, and wisdom. Divine Guru is the Philosopher's Store — touching it, one is transformed. Divine Guru is the sacred shrine of pilgrimage and the pool of divine ambrosia; bathing in the Guru's Wisdom, one experiences the Infinite. Divine Guru is the Creator, and the destroyer of all sins; Divine Guru is the purifier of sinners. Divine Guru existed at the primal beginning, throughout the ages, in each and every age. Divine Guru is the mantra of the Lord's Name; chanting it, one is saved. O God, please be merciful to me, that I may be with the Divine Guru; I am a foolish sinner, but holding on to Him, I am carried across. Divine Guru is the True Guru, the supreme Lord God, the transcendent Lord; Nanak bows in humble reverence to the Lord, the Divine Guru." Bibiji Inderjit Kaur, *Mantra: Personal Guidance Through the Power of the Word*, 2016; p.252-253.

(In the original class, the recording
"Guru Dev Mata Guru Dev Pita" by
Guru Jiwan Singh was played.)

Guroo Dayv Maataa Guroo
Dayv Pitaa Gurdayv
Suaamee Paramaysuraa
Guroo Dayv Sakhaa Agiaan
Bhanjan Guroo Dayv
Bandhip Sahodaraa
Guroo Dayv Daataa Har
Naam Updaysai Guroo
Dayv Mant Nirodharaa
Guroo Dayv Saant Sat Budh Moorat
Guroo Dayv Paaras Paras Paraa
Guroo Dayv Teerath Amrit Sarovar
Gur Giaan Majan Aparanparaa
Guroo Dayv Kartaa Sabh
Paap Hartaa Guroo Dayv
Patit Pavit Karaa
Guroo Dayv Aad Jugaad Jug Jug
Guroo Dayv Mant Har Jap Udharaa
Guroo Dayv Sangat Prabh
Mayl Kar Kirpaa Hum Moor
Paapee Kit Lag Tara
Guroo Dayv Satgur Parabhram
Parmaysar Guroo Dayv
Naanak Har Namaskaraa

8) **Self-Massage.** Sit and vigorously
massage every part of your body.
Continue for **2 ½ minutes**.

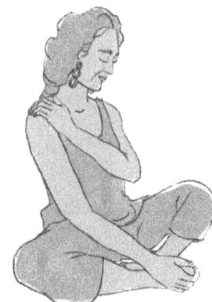

(25) Total Body Engagement Routine

July 1, 1994

There are no breaks between exercises, unless indicated.

1) **Wide Leg Lifts.** Lie on the back, stretch the arms straight out to the sides on the ground, and open the legs wide on the ground. Lift the legs up to 90 degrees and bring them back down. Keep the legs straight and continue for **1 minute**. *If doing this exercise in a group, hold the hand of the person on either side.*

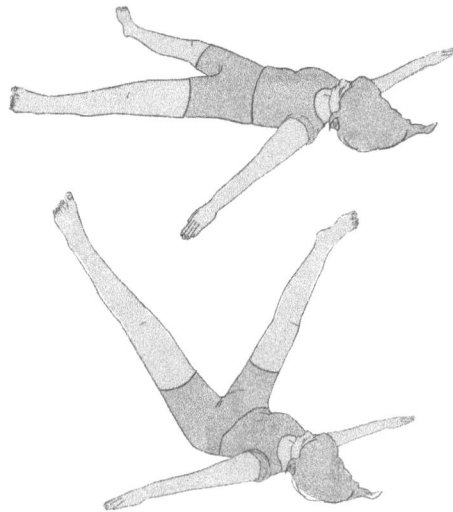

2) **Wide-Leg Sit-Ups.** Remain on the ground in the posture. Sit up, keeping the legs open and the arms stretched to the sides, then lie back down. Continue for **1 ½ minutes**. *If doing this exercise in a group, hold the hand of the person on either side and move in unison.*

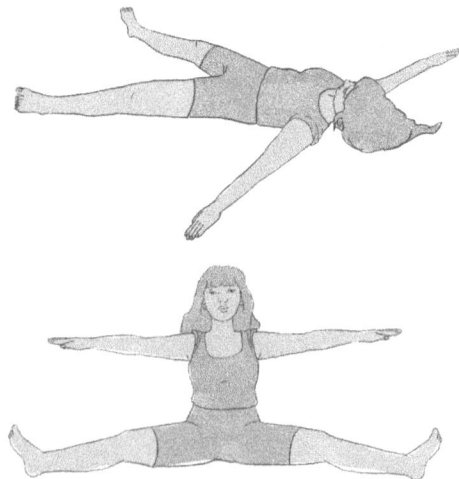

3) Wide-Leg Lifts and Sit-Ups.
Remain on the ground in the posture
and raise both the torso and the legs (as
in exercises 1 and 2) to form a V shape.
Keep the legs open and straight and the
arms stretched out to the sides, then
lie back down. Continue for **1 minute**.
*If doing this exercise in a group,
hold the hand of the person on
either side and move in unison.*

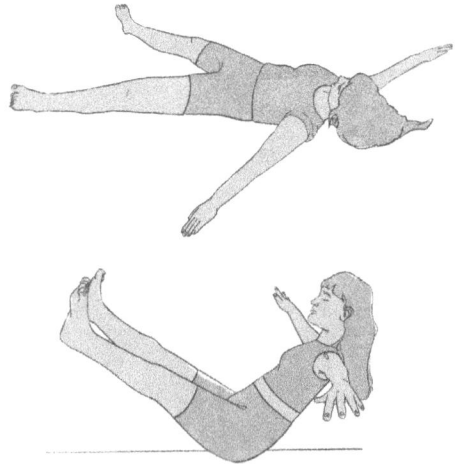

4) Traveling Sitting Jumps. Sit in
Easy Pose with the hands interlaced
on top of the head. Push from
the lower legs and jump the body
backward several times, then jump
forward several times. Continue
to jump and travel backward and
forward alternately for **1 ½ minutes**.

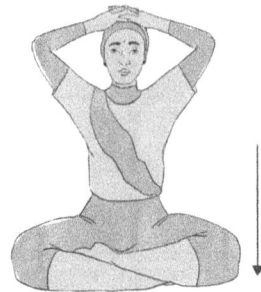

5) Bhangra Dance. Stand up and
dance to the beat. Keep the arms
raised above the Heart Center, move
the shoulders up and down, and
shift the weight from one foot to the
other so that one foot is always off
the ground. Continue for **9 minutes**.
(In the original class, Punjabi Drums
were played to keep the rhythm.)

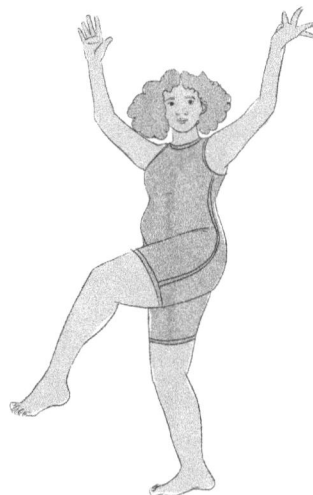

continue on next page »

6) **Front Kick Dance.** a) Stand straight and place the hands on the hips. Swing one leg up forward parallel to the ground, and down as the other leg swings up. Continue hopping from one foot to the other. Move in rhythm (one kick per second) for **5 minutes**. b) Raise the arms up above shoulder level and use them to balance the movement of the legs. Continue in a steady rhythm for **2 minutes**. (In the original class, Punjabi Drums were played to keep the rhythm.)

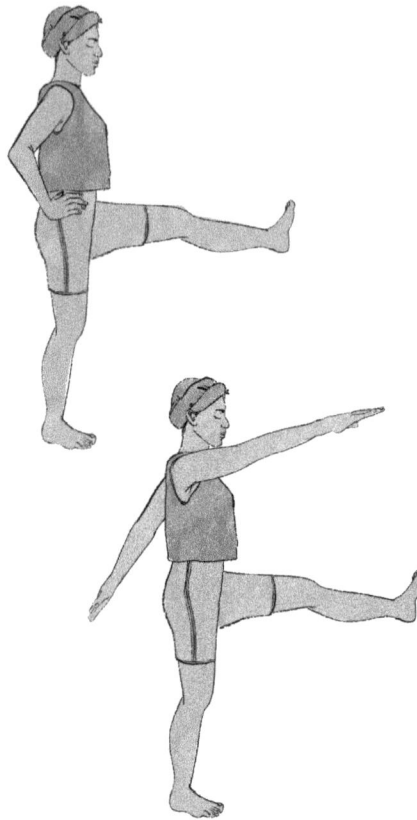

7) **Lotus Meditation.** Sit in Easy Pose with a straight spine and apply a light Neck Lock. Hold the hands in front of the Heart Center and join the base of the hands and the tips of the thumbs and Mercury (little) fingers with space between the palms and the other fingers spread apart in Lotus Mudra. Close the eyes and focus on the chin. Chant **HAR** and pull the Navel Point in with each repetition. Consolidate and receive the virtues

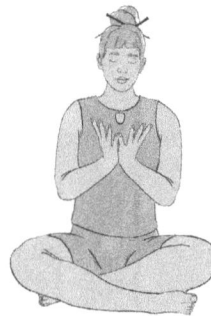

of the five elements[8] through the lotus. Continue for **6 minutes**. (In the original class, the recording "Tantric Har" by Simran Kaur was played.)
Chant so the tip of the tongue works with the navel, and the open Lotus Mudra integrates the earth and heavens, self and spirit, just like the lotus flower is elevated with its roots in the mud.

8) **Bhangra Dance**. Stand up and dance to the music. Keep the arms raised above the Heart Center, move the shoulders up and down, and shift the weight from one foot to the other so that one foot is always off the ground. Continue for **4 minutes**. (In the original class, Bhangra music was played.)
If doing this exercise in a group, hold hands and dance with a partner.

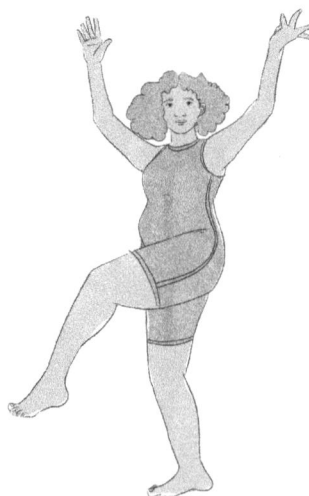

---

8   The five elements and their qualities are: earth, steadiness; water, creativity and affection; fire, purification; air, hope and forgiveness; ether, command, honor and contentment.

continue on next page »

9) **Sit in the Sun.** Sit in Easy Pose
with a straight spine and a light Neck
Lock facing the sun. Relax the elbows
by the sides, bring the forearms
up, and angle the palms toward the
sun. Close the eyes and let the sun
shine on the eyelids and forehead.
Chant **GURDAYV MAATAA
GURDAYV PITAA**[9] for **17 minutes**.
(In the original class, the recording
"Guru Dev Mata Guru Dev Pita" by
Guru Jiwan Singh was played.)
TO END: Inhale deeply and
suspend the breath, then exhale.
Repeat this cycle 2 more times.

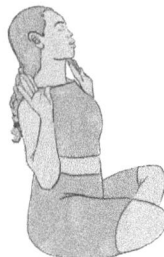

9   This mantra translates as "Divine Guru is my
mother, Divine Guru is my father; Divine Guru is my
transcendent Lord and Master. Divine Guru is my
companion, the destroyer of ignorance; Divine Guru is
my relative and brother. Divine Guru is the Giver, the
Teacher of the Lord's Name. Divine Guru is the mantra
which never fails. Divine guru is the image of peace,
truth, and wisdom. Divine Guru is the Philosopher's
Store — touching it, one is transformed. Divine Guru
is the sacred shrine of pilgrimage, and the pool of
divine ambrosia; bathing in the Guru's Wisdom, one
experiences the Infinite. Divine Guru is the Creator, and
the destroyer of all sins; Divine Guru is the purifier of
sinners. Divine Guru existed at the primal beginning,
throughout the ages, in each and every age. Divine Guru
is the mantra of the Lord's Name; chanting it, one is
saved. O God, please be merciful to me, that I may be
with the Divine Guru; I am a foolish sinner, but holding
on to Him, I am carried across. Divine Guru is the True
Guru, the supreme Lord God, the transcendent Lord;
Nanak bows in humble reverence to the Lord, the Divine
Guru." Bibiji Inderjit Kaur, *Mantra: Personal Guidance
Through the Power of the Word*, 2016; p. 252-253

Guroo Dayv Maataa Guroo
Dayv Pitaa Gurdayv
Suaamee Paramaysuraa
Guroo Dayv Sakhaa Agiaan
Bhanjan Guroo Dayv
Bandhip Sahodaraa
Guroo Dayv Daataa Har
Naam Updaysai Guroo
Dayv Mant Nirodharaa
Guroo Dayv Saant Sat Budh Moorat
Guroo Dayv Paaras Paras Paraa
Guroo Dayv Teerath Amrit Sarovar
Gur Giaan Majan Aparanparaa
Guroo Dayv Kartaa Sabh
Paap Hartaa Guroo Dayv
Patit Pavit Karaa
Guroo Dayv Aad Jugaad Jug Jug
Guroo Dayv Mant Har Jap Udharaa
Guroo Dayv Sangat Prabh
Mayl Kar Kirpaa Hum Moor
Paapee Kit Lag Tara
Guroo Dayv Satgur Parabhram
Parmaysar Guroo Dayv
Naanak Har Namaskaraa

(26) Stimulate Circulation with Leg Lift Series

July 2, 1994

There are no pauses between exercises, except when indicated.

1) **Raised Leg Balance.** a) Stand with the hands on the hips. Raise the left leg up in front of the body, parallel to the ground. Keep the leg straight and do not let it come down for **3 minutes**. b) Switch legs and hold the right leg up for **1 ½ minutes**. *When you raise the left leg, it affects the right side of the brain, and vice versa.*

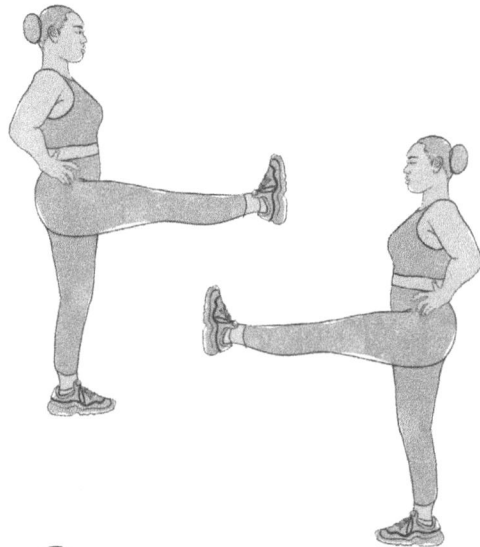

2) **Standing Leg Lifts.** Stand with the hands on the hips. Alternately raise and lower the legs. Keep the legs straight and kick upward with force. Move in rhythm for **3 ½ minutes**. (In the original class, Punjabi Drums were played to keep the rhythm.)

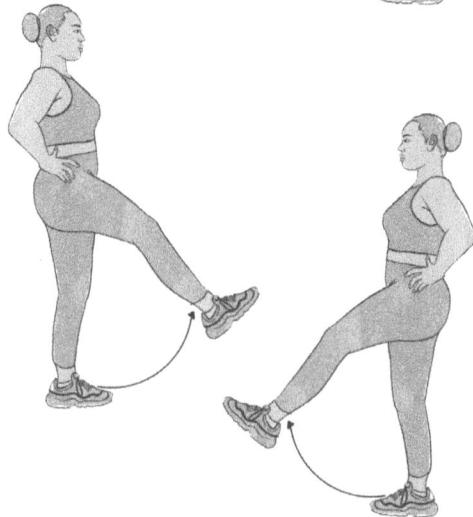

3) **Jump on All Fours.** Stand on your hands and feet with equal weight. Jump up and down so all four leave and return to the ground at the same time. Continue for **4 minutes**. (In the original class, Punjabi Drums were played to keep the rhythm.) *This exercise is good for metabolism and overeating.*

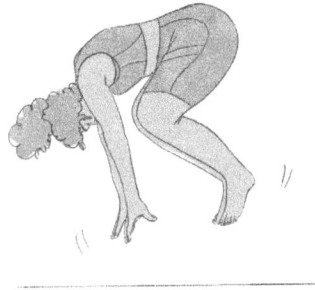

4) **Alternate Leg Lift Series**. a) Lie on the back with the fingers interlaced behind the head at the hairline and the elbows stretched out to the sides. Alternately raise each leg to 90 degrees and lower it in rhythm. Continue powerfully for **2 minutes**. b) Release the hands and bring the arms alongside the body. Alternately raise the opposite arm and leg. Continue for **30 seconds**. (In the original class, Punjabi Drums were played to keep the rhythm.)

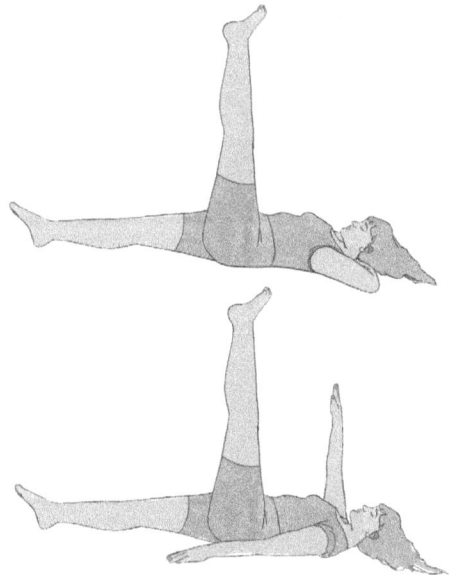

5) **Bhangra Dance.** Standing up and dance to the music. Bring the arms up and move the shoulders up and down. Hop or jump from one foot to the other so that only one foot touches the ground at a time. Move in rhythm with the music. Continue for **3 ½ minutes**. (In the original class, Punjabi Drums were played to keep the rhythm.)

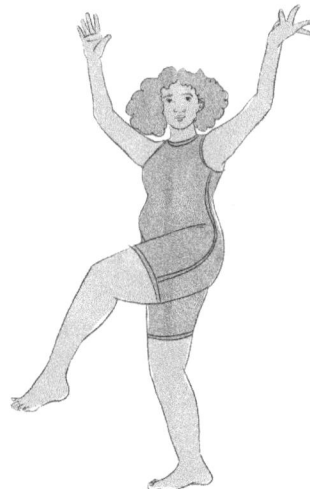

continue on next page »

6) **Parallel Forward Bend Heels Together.** Stand straight with the heels together and the toes open at a 45-degree angle. Extend the arms straight out in front of the body, palms facing down. Bend from the hips and stretch forward so that the upper body and arms are parallel to the ground. Keep the legs and spine straight. Hold the stretch for **2 ½ minutes**. Come up very slowly.

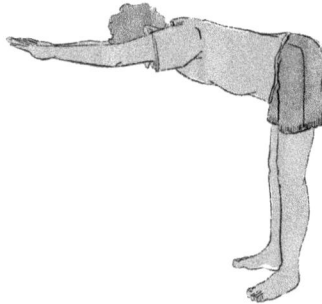

7) **Stimulate Circulation Series.** a) Stand up straight. Make fists with the hands and hit the chest with the fists. Continue for **30 seconds**. b) Hit the thighs for **10 seconds**. c) Hit the lower back and kidney area for **10 seconds**. (In the original class, Punjabi Drums were played to keep the rhythm.)

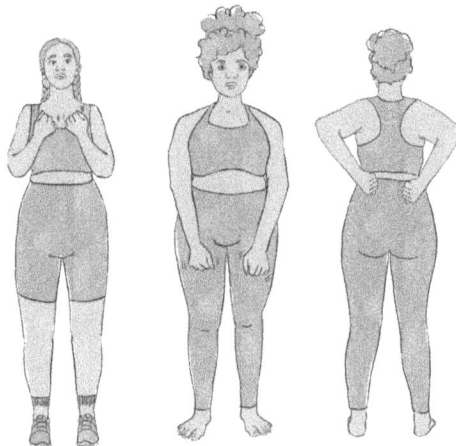

8) **Partner Wrestle.** ▲ Choose a partner, and begin to wrestle. Try to take the other person down and pin them to the ground. Continue for **1 ½ minutes**.

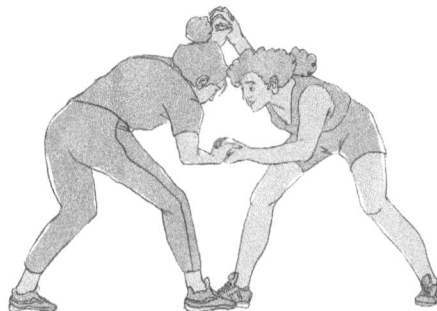

9) **Sit in the Sun.** Sit in a meditative posture, facing the sun. Open the arms wide, parallel to the ground, and bend the wrists back slightly so that the palms open outward. Close the eyes and let the sun shine on the eyelids and forehead. Meditate and sing with the music. Continue for **4 ½ minutes**. (In the original class, uplifting music was played.)

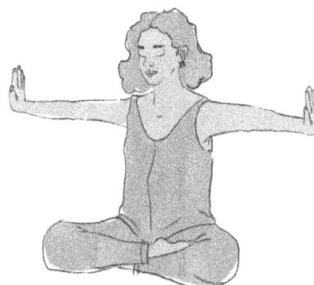

(27) Pelvic Tilt Dance Groove

Alternative:
Diaphragm Dance Party
July 3, 1994

There are no pauses between exercises.

1) **Standing Side Bends With Crossed Arms.** Stand straight, feet hip-width apart, and cross the arms on the chest, firmly grasping the opposite shoulders. Bend the whole spine to the left, then bend all the way to the right. Continue alternating for **1 ½ minutes**.

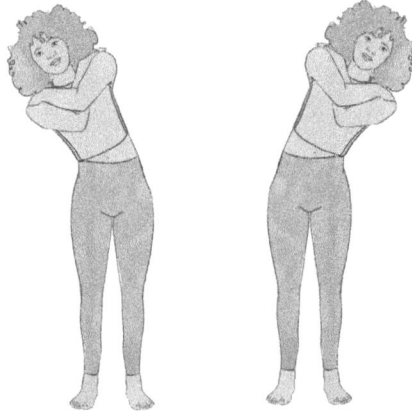

2) **Fly Up.** From standing, jump up, forcefully throwing the arms and legs wide in the air. Continue for **4 minutes**. *This exercise stretches and opens the diaphragm.*

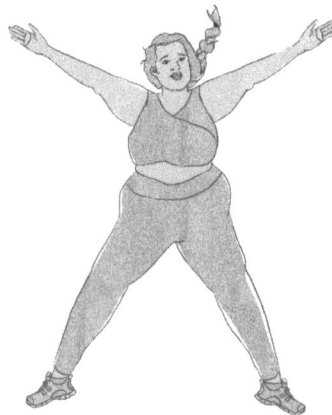

KRI KUNDALINI RESEARCH INSTITUTE

3) **Bhangra Dance.** a) Stand up and dance to the music. Keep the arms raised above the head, and move the shoulders up and down. Move the body in rhythm with the music and shift the weight from one foot to the other so that one foot is always off the ground. Continue for **4 minutes**. (In the original class, Bhangra music was played.) b) Continue to dance with the arms and hands raised, move the shoulders, and flex the upper rib cage for **4 minutes**. (In the original class, Punjabi Drums were played to keep the rhythm.)

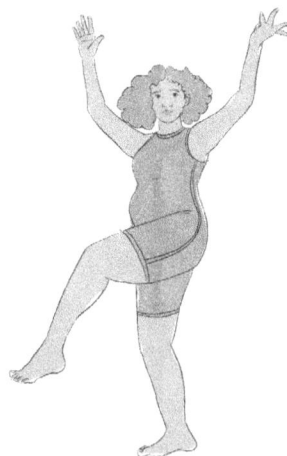

4) **Bowing Series.** a) Sit in Easy Pose with a straight spine and the arms stretched straight up. Bend forward from the hips, bringing the palms and forehead to the ground in front of you, and come back up. Move rhythmically (2 seconds per cycle) for **1 ½ minutes**. b) Remain sitting and stretch the legs wide apart. Continue to bend forward, touching the ground with the palms and forehead, for **30 seconds**. c) Remain sitting with the legs open wide and interlace the fingers behind the small of the back. Continue to bend forward, touching the ground with the forehead, and lifting the arms as high as possible for **30 seconds**.

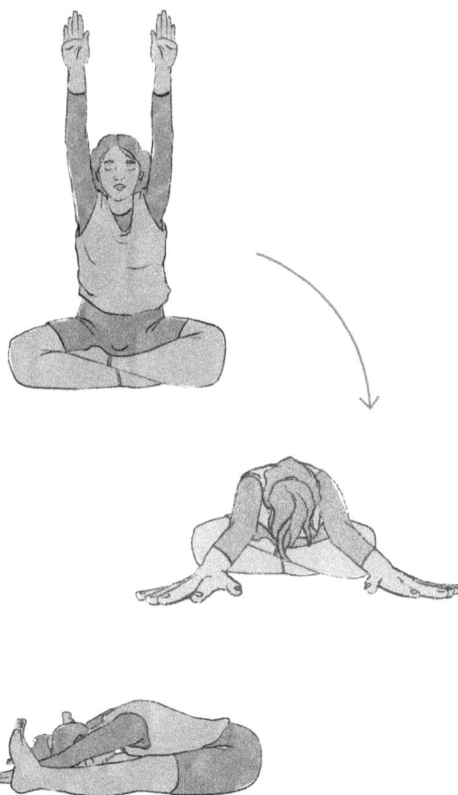

continue on next page »

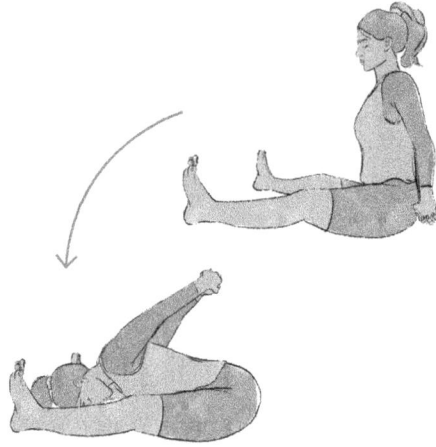

5) Body Drops. Sit with the legs together straight forward and the palms on the ground beside the hips. Push up on the hands, keeping the back straight, lift the body up, and drop back down. Continue at a quick pace (1 cycle per second) for **1 minute**.

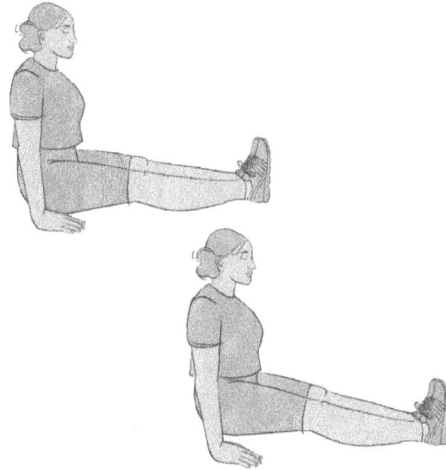

6) Sit-Up Forward Stretch. Lie down on the back with the arms on the ground overhead. Sit up and touch the toes with the hands, using the core. Return to the starting position and continue for **2 minutes**, moving as quickly as possible for the second minute. *Engage the core strongly before moving, and bend the knees, if necessary, to avoid overtaxing the hip flexors.*

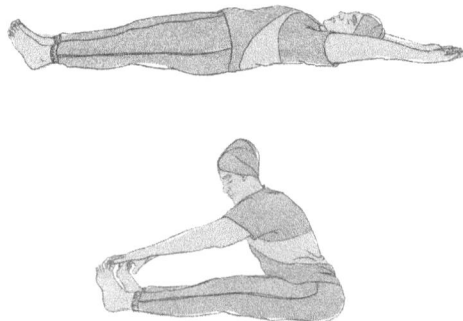

7) **Double Leg Lifts.** Lie down on the back with the arms on the ground overhead. Raise both legs up to 90 degrees and bring them down. Keep the legs straight and the feet together. Continue at a moderate pace (2 seconds per cycle) for **1 ½ minutes**.

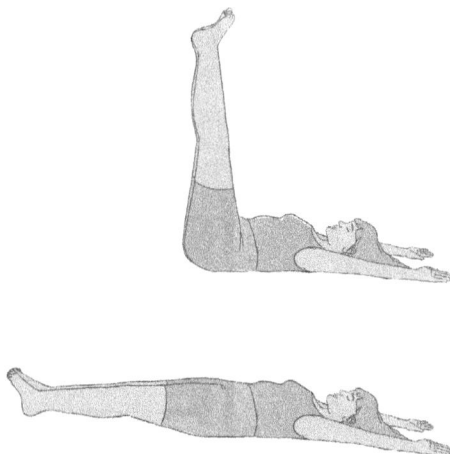

8) **Pelvic Tilt Dance.** Stand with the feet shoulder-width apart and the knees slightly bent, hands on the waist. Tilt the pelvis forward and backward. Dance and shake the pelvis quickly and rhymically for **6 minutes**. (In the original class, Punjabi Drums were played to keep the rhythm.)

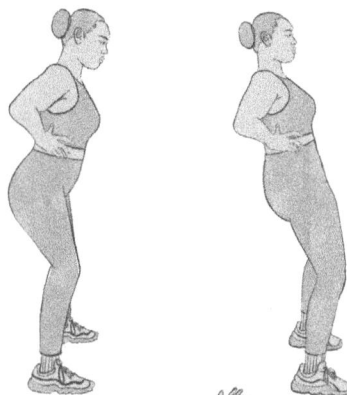

9) **Dance Party.** Dance to the music gracefully and vigorously for **13 minutes**. (In the original class, upbeat music was played and various cultural dance styles were led.)

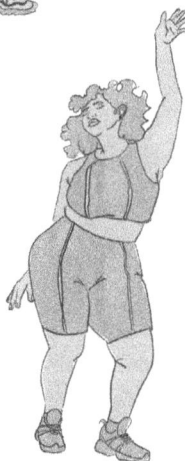

continue on next page »

10) **Crow Squat Series.** a) Stand with the feet together and extend the arms straight out to the sides. Squat down and come back up, keeping the arms straight and using the strength of your outstretched arms to pull yourself up. Continue for **1 minute**. b) Interlace the hands on top of the head and continue for **30 seconds**. c) Interlock the hands behind the back and continue for **30 seconds**.

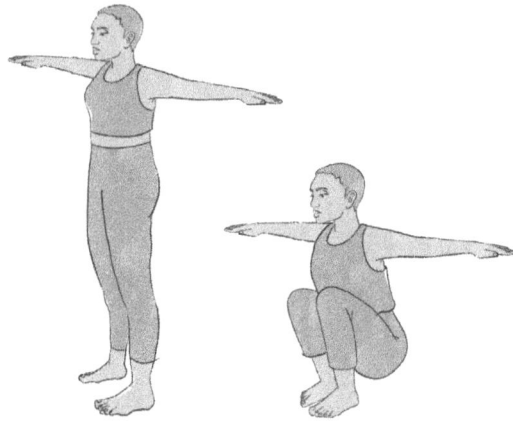

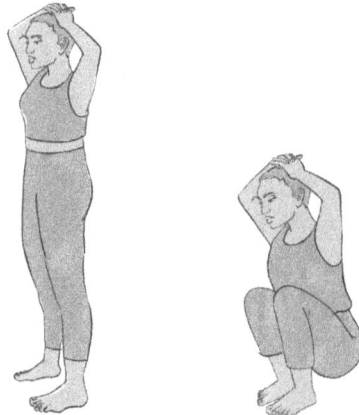

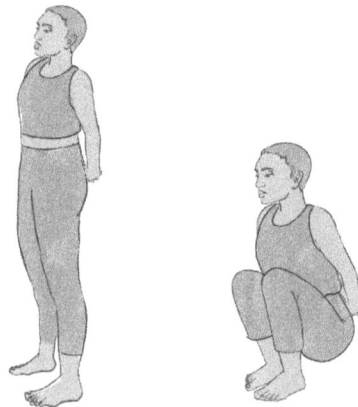

11) **Partner Wrestle.** ▲ Choose a partner, and begin to wrestle. Try to take the other person down and pin them to the ground. Continue for **1 minute**.

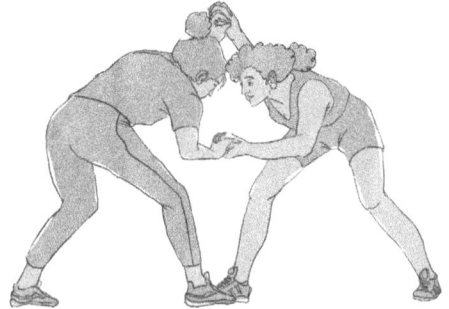

12) **Sit in the Sun with Concentration.** a) Sit in Easy Pose with a straight spine and a light Neck Lock facing the sun. Relax the elbows by the sides, bring the forearms up, and angle the palms toward the sun. Close the eyes, focus on the chin, and let the sun shine on the eyelids and forehead. Meditate and concentrate through the distraction of the music. Continue for **2 minutes**. (In the original class, loud and discordant music was played.) b) Maintain the posture and chant **HAR** once per second. Pull the Navel Point with each repetition. Continue for **2 minutes**. (In the original class, Tantric Har by Sirman Kaur was played to keep the rhythm.) c) Maintain the posture and sing with the music. Continue for **4 minutes**. (In the original class, uplifting music was played.) TO END: Inhale deeply and exhale three times.

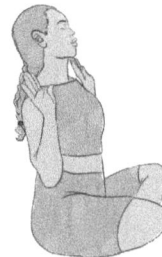

13) **Chant and Hold Hands.** Close the eyes and sing with the music from the Navel Point. Continue for **3 minutes**. (In the original class, the recording "Sat Nam Ji" by Bibi Amarjit Kaur was played.) *If doing this exercise in a group, sit in lines and hold hands with the person on either side.*

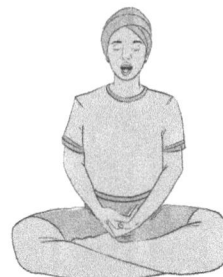

(28) Clear Toxins and Stimulate the Circulatory System

July 4, 1994

There are no pauses between exercises.

1) **Crow Squats With Diagonal Arms.** Stand straight and extend the arms out to the sides, palms facing down. Hold the right arm at 60 degrees above parallel and the left arm at 60 degrees below parallel. Squat down, then immediately bounce back up. Keep the spine straight and the arms in position. Start slowly to find the angle and hold your balance, and continue (2 seconds per cycle) for **3 minutes**. *Have no thoughts; be alert, cautious, and meditative to keep your balance.*

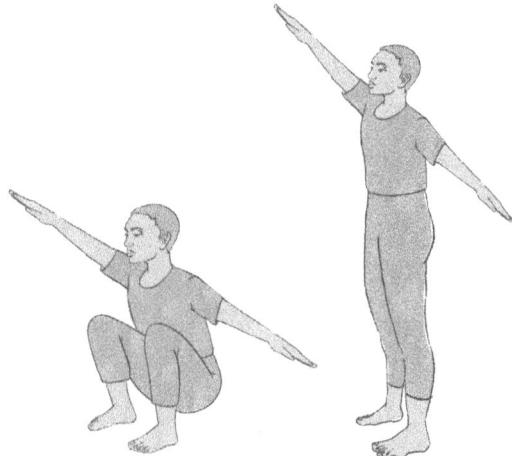

2) **Jump On All Fours.** Stand on your hands and feet with equal weight. Jump up and down so all four leave and return to the ground at the same time. Continue for **2 minutes**.

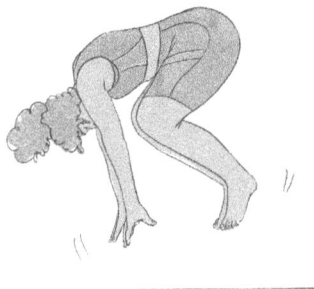

170

3) **Sitting Jumps.** Sit in Easy Pose with the hands interlocked behind the small of the back. Jump the sit bones up and down for **2 minutes**. *This exercise stimulates the metabolism and clears sluggishness.*

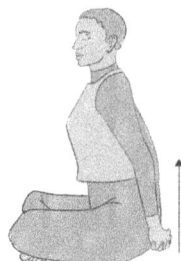

4) **Hit the Chest With Knees.** Lie on the back. Hold both legs up at 60 degrees and alternately bring the knees in to hit the chest. Move fast (2 hits per second) and continue for **2 ½ minutes**. *Bring up any anger and release it. You may yell and scream.*

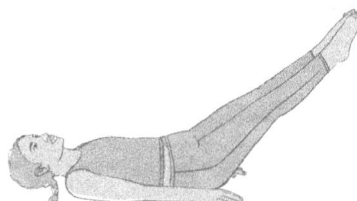

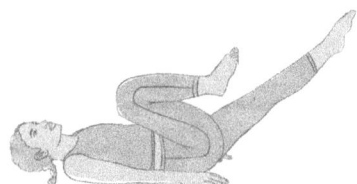

5) **Bhangra Dance.** Stand up and dance to the music. Cross and uncross the wrists in front of the Heart Center as you move in rhythm with the music. Hop from one foot to the other so that only one foot touches the ground at a time. Continue for **3 ½ minutes**. (In the original class, Bhangra music was played.) *This is great exercise for your heart, diaphragm, and brain.*

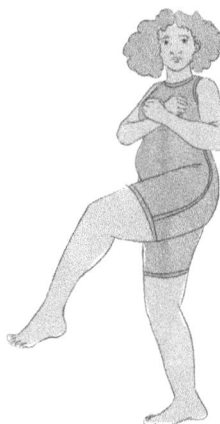

continue on next page »

6) **Arm Circle Series.** a) Stand straight with the feet shoulder-width apart. Interlock the hands together in front of the body with the arms straight. Moving from the shoulders, make as large a circle as possible with the hands. Keep the arms straight and move fast and powerfully. Let the whole body get into it and continue for **1 minute**. b) Make fists and alternately rotate the arms in large backward circles. Let the weight of the fist build momentum. Keep the arms straight and move fast for **1 minute**. c) Circle both arms backward in unison. Move powerfully for **2 ½ minutes**.

Move with force to stimulate the circulatory system and clear toxins from the upper body.

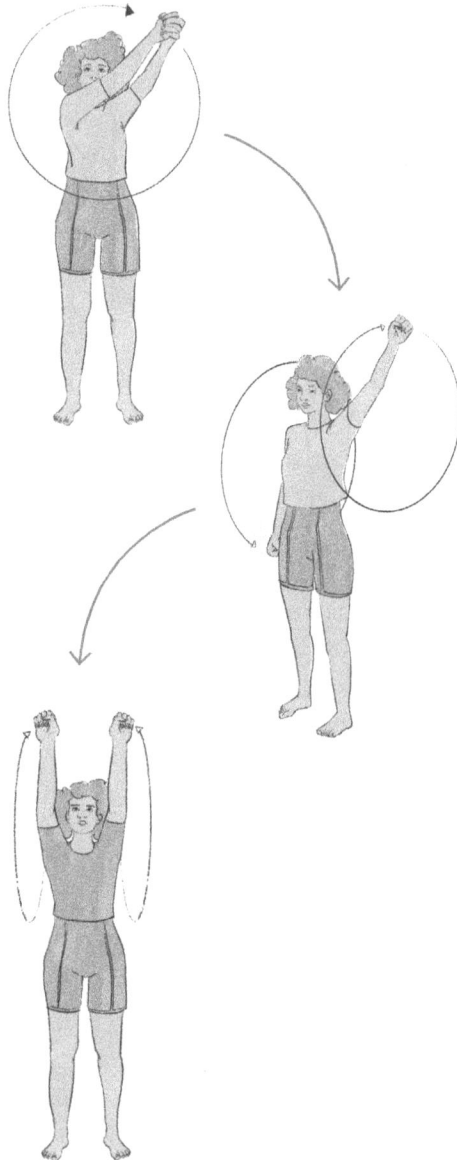

7) **Partner Wrestle.** ▲ Choose a partner, and begin to wrestle. Try to take the other person down and pin them to the ground. Continue for **3 minutes**.

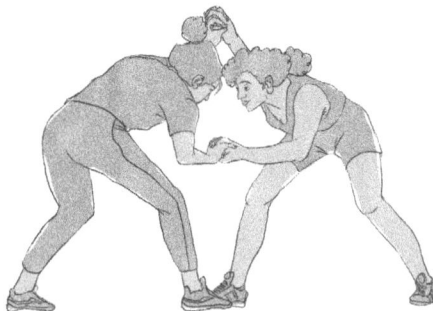

8) **Free Dance.** Dance freely to the music. Move the body vigorously. Continue for **3 ½ minutes**. (In the original class, Bhangra music was played.)

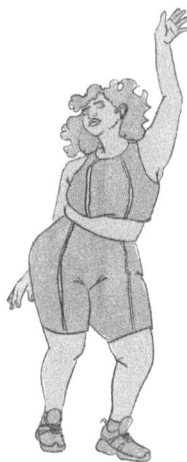

(29) Total Body Activation Sequence

July 5, 1994

There are no pauses between exercises.

1) **Full Body Flex.** Stand straight with the feet shoulder-width apart and place the hands on the hips. Undulate and flex the entire body, from your toes to the top of the head. The pelvis will move forward and backward. Continue for **2 ½ minutes**.

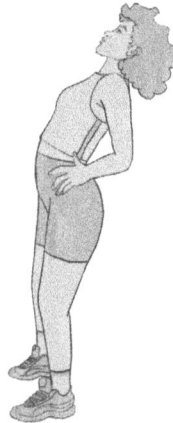

2) **Forward Bend With Arm Swings.** Stand with the feet shoulder-width apart. Bend forward, with the upper body parallel to the ground and the arms hanging down. Keep the legs and spine straight and look forward. Swing both arms together in an arc from left to right. Move powerfully so that the body twists with the movement. Continue for **1 ½ minutes**.

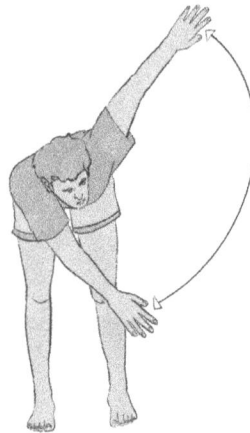

KRI KUNDALINI RESEARCH INSTITUTE

3) Crow Squats with Hand Lock.
Stand straight with the feet shoulder-width apart. Interlock the hands overhead and stretch the arms straight up. Squat down in Crow Pose and come back up. Use the strength of the Navel Point to come up with force for **1 ½ minutes**.

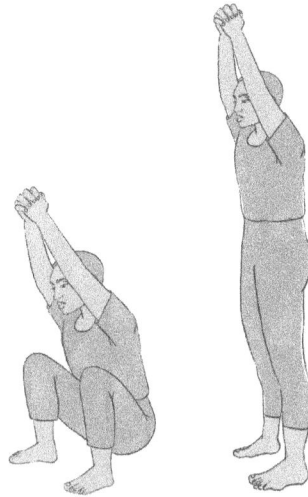

4) Belly Jumps. Lie on the stomach and interlock the hands at the base of the spine. Jump up and down, lifting the body off the ground. Continue at a steady pace for **3 ½ minutes**.

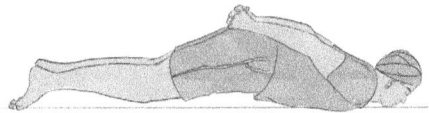

5) Rocking Chair. Remain on the stomach with the hands interlocked. Rock powerfully forward so the legs come off the ground, and back powerfully so the upper body comes off the ground. Keep the legs straight and continue for **1 minute**.

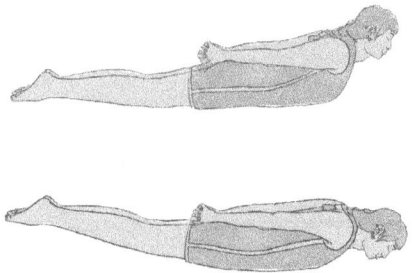

6) Erratic Movement. Sit in Easy Pose. Place the hands on the Navel Center, one on top of the other. Keeping the legs and hips on the ground, move the rest of the body in a wild, erratic manner without pattern or rhythm for **1 minute**.

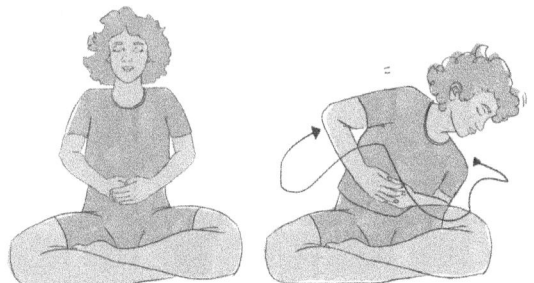

continue on next page »

7) **Lion Roar.** Stand on the hands and knees, with the hands directly under the shoulders and the knees directly under the hips. Roar like a lion loudly for **1 minute**.

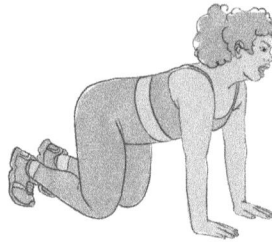

8) **Bhangra Dance.** Stand up and dance to the music. Make fists with the hands and keep the arms up and out to the sides, above shoulder level. Hop from one foot to the other so that only one foot touches the ground at a time. Move in rhythm for **4 minutes**. Relax. *Holding the arms up in this way adjusts the magnetic field, which balances the body.*

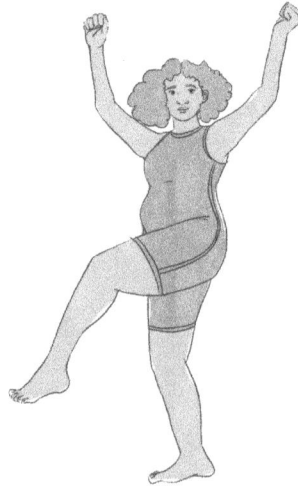

9) **Har Meditation.** Sit in Easy Pose with a straight spine and a light Neck Lock. Bring the hands up near the shoulders, elbows relaxed at the sides of the body. With the right hand, touch the tip of the thumb and the tip of the Sun (ring) finger. With the left hand, touch the tip of the thumb and the tip of the Jupiter (index) finger. Close the eyes and roll them down to focus on the chin. Chant **HAR** with the tip of the tongue for **3 ½ minutes**. (In the original class, the recording "Tantric Har" by Simran Kaur was played.)

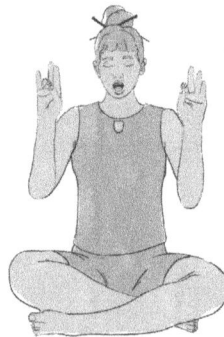

(30) Self-Esteem Workout

July 6, 1994

There are no pauses between exercises.

1) **Elbow Stretch.** Stand straight with the feet shoulder-width apart. Bring the hands up to eye level, fingertips pointing toward each other, palms facing down. The elbows relaxed out to the sides, lower than the hands. Quickly and powerfully extend both arms with a jolt straight out at eye level with no bend in the elbow or wrist. Immediately return to the starting position. Fix the eyes forward and continue for **1 ½ minutes**.

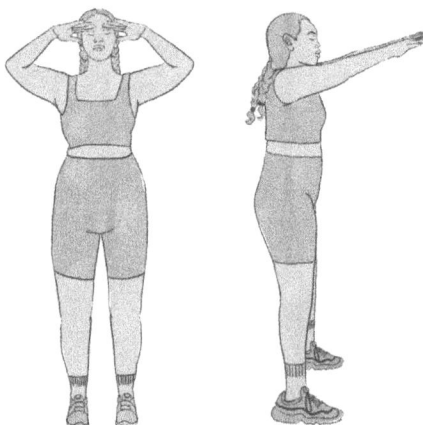

2) **Stand and Touch Ground.** Stand straight with the heels together and the feet open at a 45-degree angle. Stretch the arms straight forward with the palms facing down. Bend forward from the hips and touch the ground with both hands. Come back up, keeping the legs and arms straight and the head in alignment with the body (2 seconds per cycle). Continue for **30 seconds**.

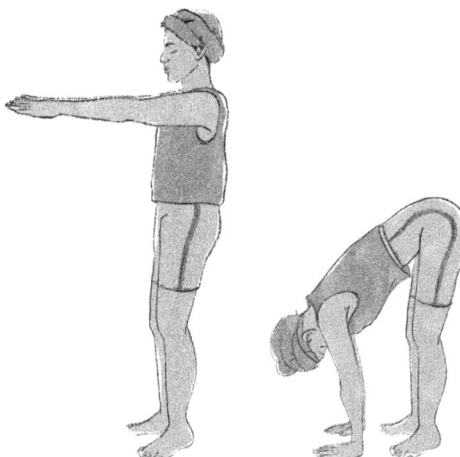

3) **Jump Up Arms Extended.** Stand straight with the feet shoulder-width apart. Stretch the arms straight up overhead. Jump up and down in a steady rhythm (1 jump per 2 seconds), keeping the arms straight. Generate the movement from the Navel Point for **2 ½ minutes**.

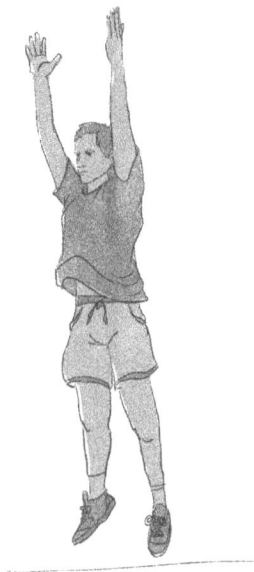

4) **Bhangra Dance.** Come standing up and dance to the music. Make fists with your hands and keep the arms up above shoulder level. Move the fists in alternate circles as you hop from one foot to the other so that only one foot touches the ground at a time. Dance vigorously for **5 minutes**. (In the original class, Bhangra music was played.)

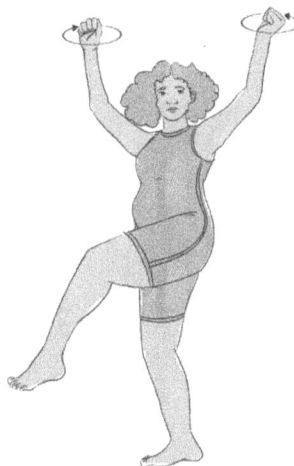

5) **Sit-Up Forward Stretch in Easy Pose.** Sit in Easy Pose. Bend forward and bring the forehead to the ground, then lay back so the back of the head touches the ground. Continue alternating between these positions in a steady fluid motion for **1 ½ minutes**.

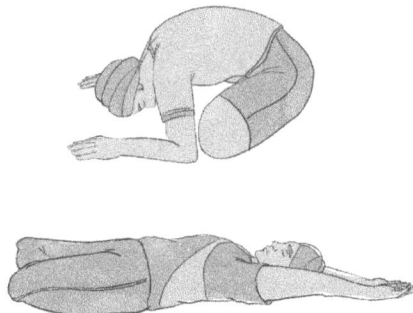

continue on next page »

6) **Bicycle Series.** a) Lie on the back and bring both legs up. Move the legs in circles alternately as if bicycling. Move fast for **30 seconds**. b) Continue the movement and circle the arms as well for **1 minute**. c) Continue both movements and roar loudly like a lion for **1 minute**.

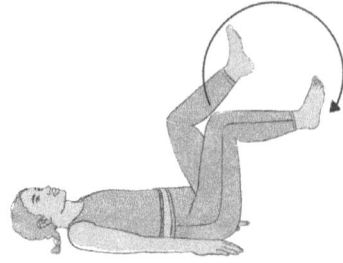

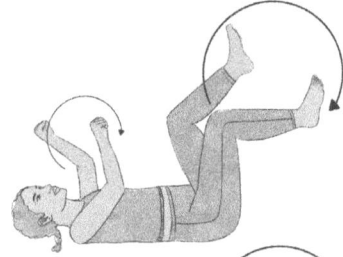

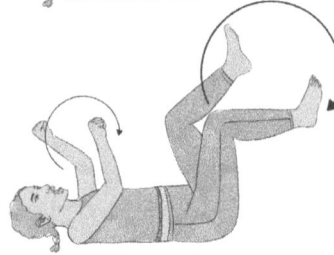

7) **Plow Pose.** a) Remain lying on the back. Bring the legs together, lift the weight onto the shoulders, and bring the feet overhead towards the ground behind you in Plow Pose. Keep the legs together and straight. Hold this position for **30 seconds**. b) Raise one leg straight up while the other leg goes down to touch the ground behind the head. Continue for **30 seconds**.

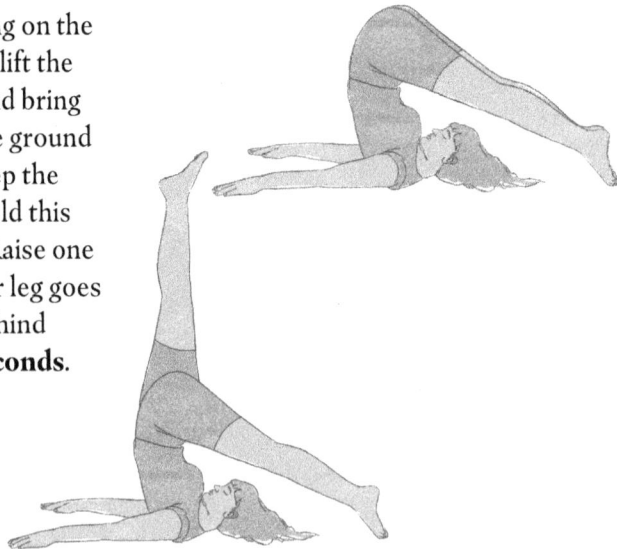

8) **Partner Wrestle.** ▲ Choose a partner, and begin to wrestle. Try to take the other person down and pin them to the ground. Continue for **1 minute**.

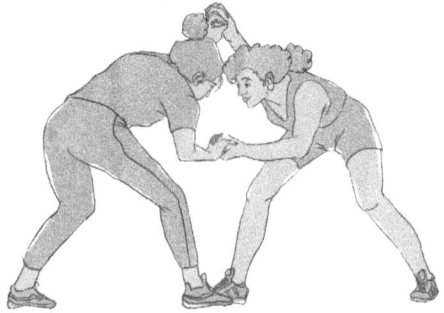

9) **Sit in the Sun.** a) Sit in Easy Pose with a straight spine and a light Neck Lock facing the sun. Relax the elbows by the sides, bring the forearms up, and angle the palms toward the sun. Close the eyes, focus at the chin, and let the sun shine on the eyelids and forehead. Continue for **3 ½ minutes**. (In the original class, uplifting music was played.) b) Remain in the posture and sing with the music for **3 minutes**. TO END: Inhale deeply, suspend briefly, and exhale. Repeat **2 more times.** Relax.
The focus on the chin activates the frontal lobe and develops intuition.

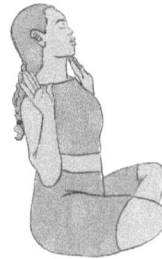

(31) Squat Series for Divine Alignment

July 7, 1994

There are no pauses between exercises.

1) **Four Step Squat Series.** Stand straight with the feet shoulder-width apart. Place the hands on the shoulders with the fingers in front and the thumbs in back, elbows out to the sides. Squat down, lay on the stomach, jump up to standing, and jump in place. Keep the hands on the shoulders throughout and repeat this sequence for **7 minutes**. *If students are doing this exercise in a group setting and need a break, the instructor may allow them to rest briefly in any of the postures.*

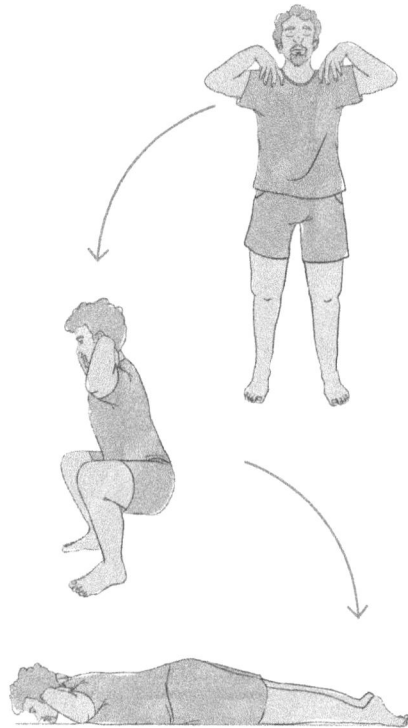

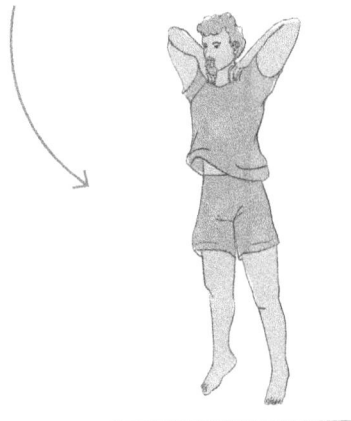

KRI KUNDALINI RESEARCH INSTITUTE

2) **Front Kick Dance.** a) Stand straight and place the hands on the hips. Swing one leg up forward parallel to the ground, and down as the other leg swings up. Continue hopping from one foot to the other. Move in rhythm (2 kicks per second) for **7 minutes**. (In the original class, Bhangra music was played.) b) Continue kicking, and with the hands in fists, move the arms back and forth in rhythm with the legs for **1 minute**. *This exercise helps clear buildup from the digestive system.*

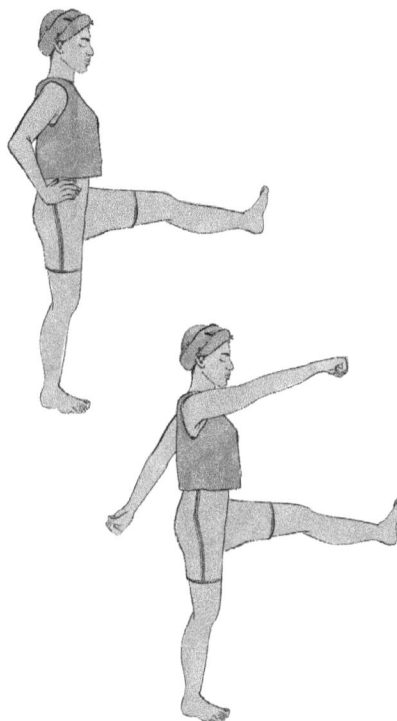

3) **I Am Affirmation.** a) Sit in Easy Pose with a straight spine and a light Neck Lock. Bring the left hand up, placing the fingertips in a vertical line in the center of the forehead, and elbow out to the side. Stretch the right arm straight forward, raise it 15 degrees above parallel to the ground, and bend the wrist so the palm faces forward. Repeat this affirmation loudly: **I AM THE LIGHT OF THE SOUL. I AM BEAUTIFUL, I AM BOUNTIFUL, I AM BLISS. I AM, I AM.** Continue for **3 minutes**. b) Remain in the

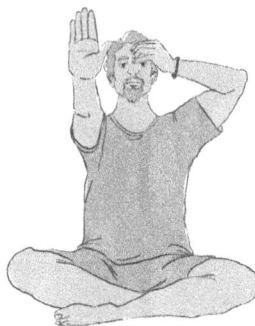

continue on next page »

posture and sing the same affirmation for **2 minutes**. c) Place the hands on the Heart Center, one on top of the other and sing with the music for **1 ½ minutes**. (In the original class, uplifting music was played.) *"God made you, you are beautiful, you are bountiful and you are blissful. Once you know that, the entire hand of nature will come to you. This is the miracle." – Yogi Bhajan*

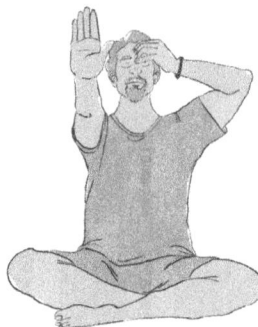

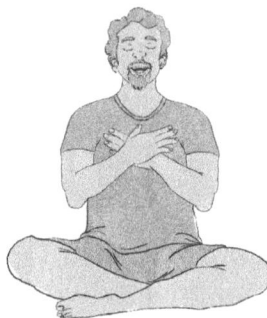

4) **Sit in the Sun.** Sit in Easy Pose with a straight spine and a light Neck Lock facing the sun. Relax the elbows by the sides, bring the forearms up, and angle the palms toward the sun. Close the eyes and let the sun shine on the eyelids and forehead. Chant **ONG NAMO GUROO DAYV NAMO** for **5 minutes**. (In the original class, the recording "Ong Namo Guru Dev Namo" by Nirinjan Kaur was played.)

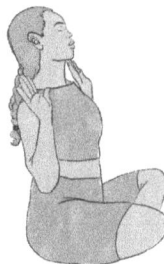

(32) For the Sake of Your Liver

July 12, 1994

There are no pauses between exercises.

1) **Jump on All Fours.** Stand on your
hands and feet with equal weight.
Jump up and down so all four leave
and return to the ground at the same
time. Use a four part rhythm with three
jumps and one pause for **1 minute**.

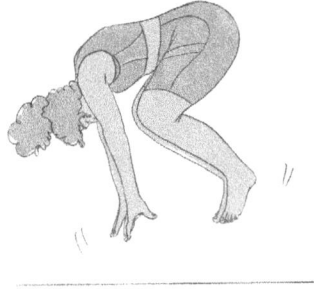

2) **Standing Leg Lifts.** Stand with the
arms straight forward and the hands
in fists, palms down. Alternately raise
and lower the legs. Keep the back
and legs straight and kick upward
with force, as high as possible.
Move in rhythm for **1 minute**.

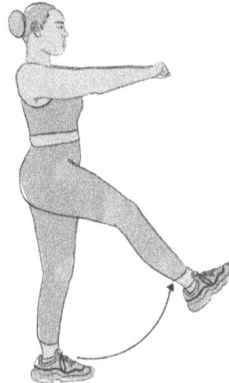

3) **Bhangra Dance.** Stand up and dance
to the music with the arms straight out
front and the hands in fists. Shift the
weight from one foot to the other so
that one foot is always off the ground.
Allow the shoulders to balance the
movement of the lower body. Continue
for **5 minutes**. (In the original class,
Bhangra music was played.)

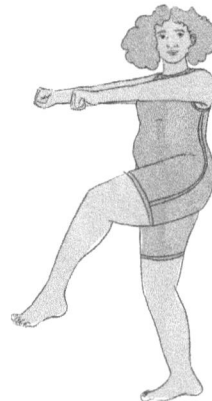

KRI KUNDALINI RESEARCH INSTITUTE

4) **Partner Wrestle.** ▲ Choose a partner, and begin to wrestle. Try to take the other person down, and pin them to the ground. Continue for **2 minutes**. Relax.

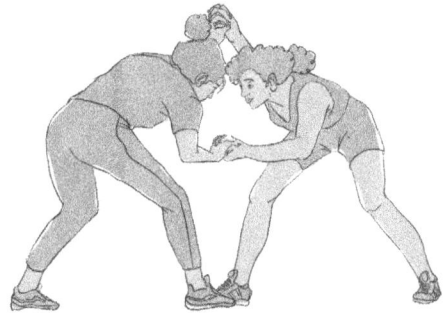

5) **Lay Flat Series.** a) Sit in Easy Pose, bend forward, and touch the forehead to the ground. b) Lay flat on the stomach. c) Return to Easy Pose. d) Lay flat on the back. Continue this series without using the hands for support, for **3 minutes**.

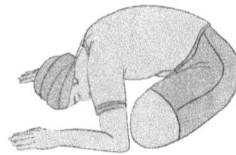

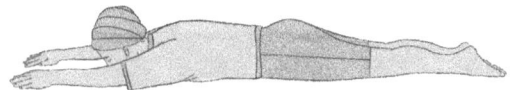

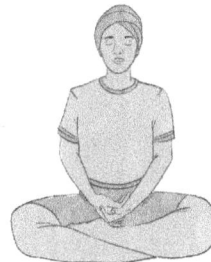

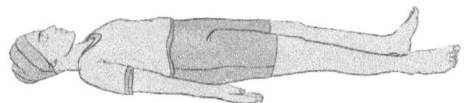

continue on next page »

6) **Rock In Bow Pose.** On the stomach, reach back and take hold of the ankles. Arch the spine and pull the body upward into Bow Pose. Rock back and forth on the stomach for **2 minutes**. TO END: Do **one repetition** of Exercise 5, Lay Flat Series.

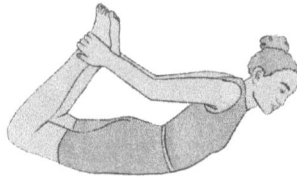

7) **Bicycle Legs in Shoulder Stand.** Lie on the back. Bend the knees in toward the chest, put the weight on the shoulders, and lift the legs up straight to come into Shoulder Stand. Place the elbows on the ground, and use the hands to support the back. Move the legs in circles alternately as if bicycling. Move quickly for **2 minutes**. TO END: Do 2 repetitions of Exercise 5, Lay Flat Series.

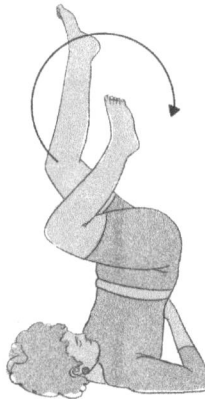

8) **Jump On All Fours Then Stand.** Stand on your hands and feet with equal weight on all four. Jump up and down so all four leave and return to the ground at the same time. Use a four part rhythm, with three jumps, then come standing up. Repeat this series for **1 ½ minutes**.

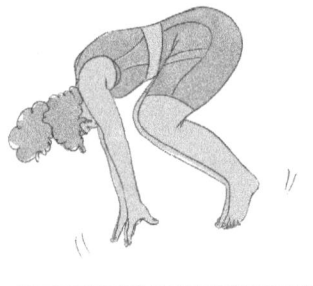

9) **Lean Back-to-Back.** Stand back to back with a partner and interlock the elbows. Close the eyes and completely relax your body. Lean into each other and let all the tension go. Hold this position for **3 minutes**. *If practicing alone, imagine you are leaning against someone's back. You may do this exercise leaning against the wall.*

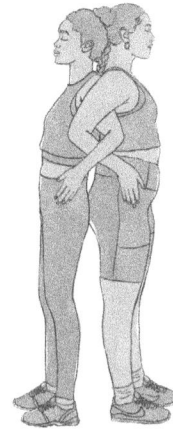

10) **Sit in the Sun.** Sit in Easy Pose with a straight spine and a light Neck Lock facing the sun. Relax the elbows by the sides, bring the forearms up, and angle the palms toward the sun. Close the eyes, focus on the chin, and let the sun shine on the eyelids and forehead. Chant **GURDAYV MAATAA GURDAYV PITAA**[10] from the heart for **15 minutes**. (In the original class, the recording "Guru Dev Mata Guru Dev Pita" by Guru Jiwan Singh was played.)

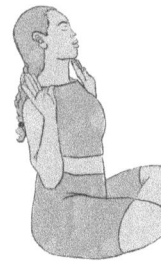

---

10 This mantra translates as "Divine Guru is my mother, Divine Guru is my father; Divine Guru is my transcendent Lord and Master. Divine Guru is my companion, the destroyer of ignorance; Divine Guru is my relative and brother. Divine Guru is the Giver, the Teacher of the Lord's Name. Divine Guru is the mantra which never fails. Divine guru is the image of peace, truth, and wisdom. Divine Guru is the Philosopher's Store — touching it, one is transformed. Divine Guru is the sacred shrine of pilgrimage, and the pool of divine ambrosia; bathing in the Guru's Wisdom, one experiences the Infinite. Divine Guru is the Creator, and the destroyer of all sins; Divine Guru is the purifier of sinners. Divine Guru existed at the primal beginning, throughout the ages, in each and every age. Divine Guru is the mantra of the Lord's Name; chanting it, one is saved. O God, please be merciful to me, that I may be with the Divine Guru; I am a foolish sinner, but holding on to Him, I am carried across. Divine Guru is the True Guru, the supreme Lord God, the transcendent Lord; Nanak bows in humble reverence to the Lord, the Divine Guru." Bibiji Inderjit Kaur, *Mantra: Personal Guidance Through the Power of the Word*, 2016; p. 252-253

Guroo Dayv Maataa Guroo
Dayv Pitaa Gurdayv
Suaamee Paramaysuraa
Guroo Dayv Sakhaa Agiaan Bhanjan
Guroo Dayv Bandhip Sahodaraa
Guroo Dayv Daataa Har
Naam Updaysai Guroo
Dayv Mant Nirodharaa
Guroo Dayv Saant Sat Budh Moorat
Guroo Dayv Paaras Paras Paraa
Guroo Dayv Teerath Amrit Sarovar
Gur Giaan Majan Aparanparaa
Guroo Dayv Kartaa Sabh
Paap Hartaa Guroo Dayv
Patit Pavit Karaa
Guroo Dayv Aad Jugaad Jug Jug
Guroo Dayv Mant Har Jap Udharaa
Guroo Dayv Sangat Prabh
Mayl Kar Kirpaa Hum Moor
Paapee Kit Lag Tara
Guroo Dayv Satgur Parabhram
Parmaysar Guroo Dayv
Naanak Har Namaskaraa

Comments: All of these exercises
stimulate the liver's metabolism, so
its functions of holding and releasing
are more balanced, allowing you to
flow with the natural rhythms of your
life. There are many substances we
encounter in modern life that adversely
affect this flow, and we may hold
onto old patterns and hidden anger.

③③ Vitality and Core Strengthening Series

July 13, 1994

There are no pauses between exercises.

1) **Bhangra Dance.** Stand up and dance to the music. Keep the arms raised above the Heart Center, move the shoulders up and down, and shift the weight from one foot to the other so that one foot is always off the ground. Continue for **10 minutes.** (In the original class, Bhangra music was played.)
If doing this exercise in a group, hold hands and dance with a partner.

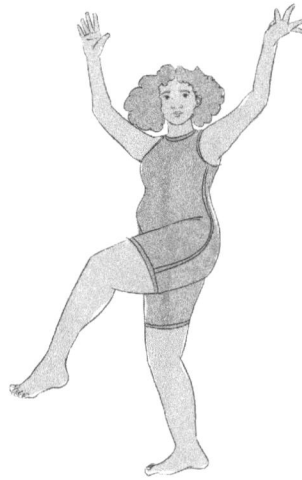

2) **Push-Up Series.** a) Come into Front Plank supporting the body on the fists and the toes. Keep the back straight and the body in alignment. Do **10 push-ups** in this posture. b) Remain in Front Plank with the hands wider than the shoulders and palms flat on the ground, fingers spread wide. Do **10 push-ups** in this posture. c) Remain in Front Plank on the fingertips. Do **10 push-ups** in this posture. d) Remain in

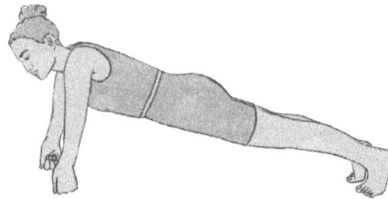

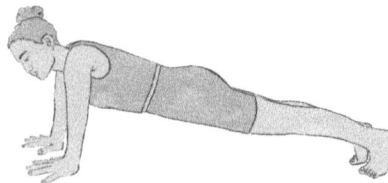

Front Plank with the hands flat on the ground and pointing back toward the toes. Do **10 push-ups** in this posture. *It is advisable to warm up your wrists before beginning this series. If you have wrist issues, keep the hands in fists for all parts of this series.*

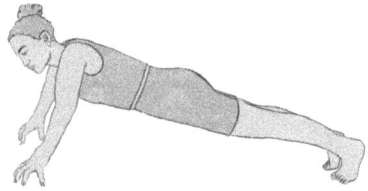

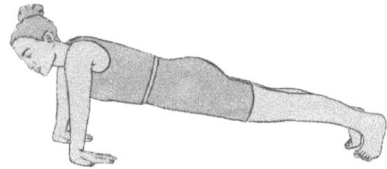

3) **Bhangra Dance.** Stand up and dance to the music. Keep the arms raised above the Heart Center, move the shoulders up and down, and shift the weight from one foot to the other so that one foot is always off the ground. Continue for **1 ½ minutes**. (In the original class, Bhangra music was played.) *If doing this exercise in a group, hold hands and dance with a partner.*

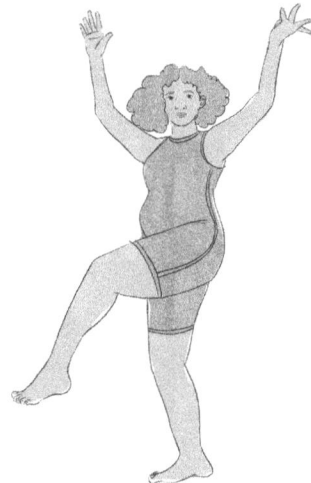

4) **Sit in the Sun.** Sit in Easy Pose with a straight spine and a light Neck Lock facing the sun. Relax the elbows by the sides, bring the forearms up, and angle the palms toward the sun. Close the eyes and let the sun shine on the eyelids and forehead. Release doubt and project yourself into Infinity for **8 minutes**. (In the original class, the recording "Meditation" by Wah! was played.)

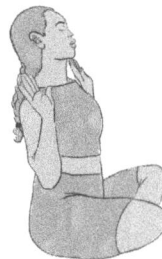

(34) Awakening and Strengthening the Spine

July 14, 1994

There are no pauses between exercises.

1) **Side-to-Side Rolls.** Lie on the back with the arms by the sides. Roll on the torso and legs from left to right, without rolling onto the stomach. Keep the legs and arms straight. Continue at a pace of 2 seconds per cycle for **4 minutes**. *This is an excellent exercise for your spine and can even be done in bed.*

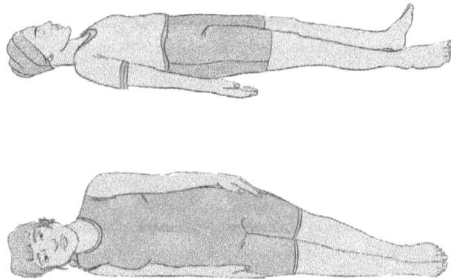

2) **Fish Out of Water.** Lie on the stomach and stretch the arms forward. Raise the arms and legs up off the ground and move like a fish out of water. Jump erratically and flop around for **2 ½ minutes**.

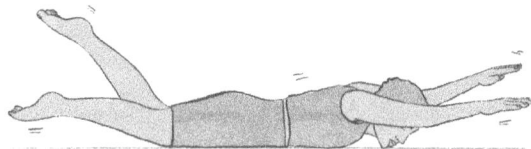

3) **Bhangra Dance.** Stand up and dance to the music. Keep the arms raised above the Heart Center, move the shoulders up and down, and shift the weight from one foot to the other so that one foot is always off the ground. Close your eyes, concentrate, and coordinate your mind and body. Dance for **8 ½ minutes**. (In the original class, Bhangra music was played.)

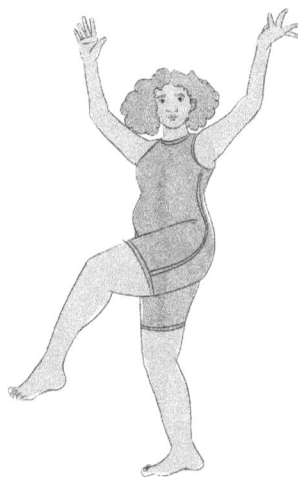

4) **Partner Wrestle.** ▲ Choose a partner, and begin to wrestle. Try to take the other person down, and pin them to the ground. Continue for **1-2 minutes**.

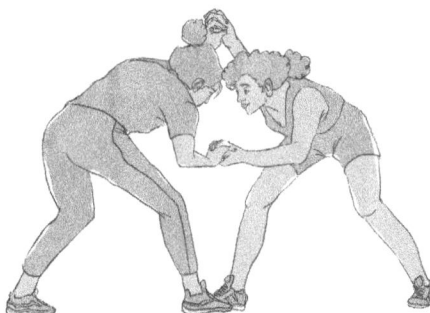

continue on next page »

5) **Sit in the Sun.** Sit in Easy Pose with a straight spine and a light Neck Lock facing the sun. Relax the elbows by the sides, bring the forearms up, and angle the palms toward the sun. Close the eyes and let the sun shine on the eyelids and forehead. Chant **GURDAYV MAATAA GURDAYV PITAA**[11] and meditate for **22 minutes**. (In the original class, the recording "Guru Dev Mata, Guru Dev Pita" by Guru Jiwan Singh was played.)

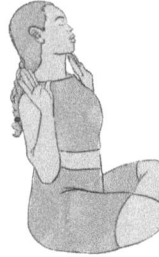

11 This mantra translates as "Divine Guru is my mother, Divine Guru is my father; Divine Guru is my transcendent Lord and Master. Divine Guru is my companion, the destroyer of ignorance; Divine Guru is my relative and brother. Divine Guru is the Giver, the Teacher of the Lord's Name. Divine Guru is the mantra which never fails. Divine guru is the image of peace, truth, and wisdom. Divine Guru is the Philosopher's Store — touching it, one is transformed. Divine Guru is the sacred shrine of pilgrimage, and the pool of divine ambrosia; bathing in the Guru's Wisdom, one experiences the Infinite. Divine Guru is the Creator, and the destroyer of all sins; Divine Guru is the purifier of sinners. Divine Guru existed at the primal beginning, throughout the ages, in each and every age. Divine Guru is the mantra of the Lord's Name; chanting it, one is saved. O God, please be merciful to me, that I may be with the Divine Guru; I am a foolish sinner, but holding on to Him, I am carried across. Divine Guru is the True Guru, the supreme Lord God, the transcendent Lord; Nanak bows in humble reverence to the Lord, the Divine Guru." Bibiji Inderjit Kaur, *Mantra: Personal Guidance Through the Power of the Word*, 2016; p. 252-253

Guroo Dayv Maataa Guroo
Dayv Pitaa Gurdayv
Suaamee Paramaysuraa
Guroo Dayv Sakhaa Agiaan
Bhanjan Guroo Dayv
Bandhip Sahodaraa
Guroo Dayv Daataa Har
Naam Updaysai Guroo
Dayv Mant Nirodharaa
Guroo Dayv Saant Sat Budh Moorat
Guroo Dayv Paaras Paras Paraa
Guroo Dayv Teerath Amrit Sarovar
Gur Giaan Majan Aparanparaa
Guroo Dayv Kartaa Sabh
Paap Hartaa Guroo Dayv
Patit Pavit Karaa
Guroo Dayv Aad Jugaad Jug Jug
Guroo Dayv Mant Har Jap Udharaa
Guroo Dayv Sangat Prabh
Mayl Kar Kirpaa Hum Moor
Paapee Kit Lag Tara
Guroo Dayv Satgur Parabhram
Parmaysar Guroo Dayv
Naanak Har Namaskaraa

(35) Navel Activation with Tantric Har

July 15, 1994

There are no pauses between exercises.

1) **Standing Torso Rotation.** Stand straight with the feet shoulder-width apart and the hands on the hips. Rotate the torso in wide circles in either direction. Move quickly for **2 minutes**. For the last minute, use your anger to roar loudly like a lion.

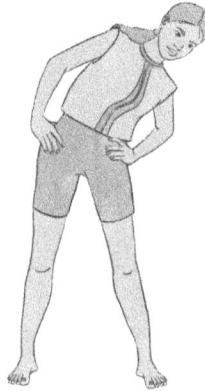

2) **Partner Wrestle.** ▲ Choose a partner, and begin to wrestle. Try to take the other person down, and pin them to the ground. Continue for **1 ½ minutes**.

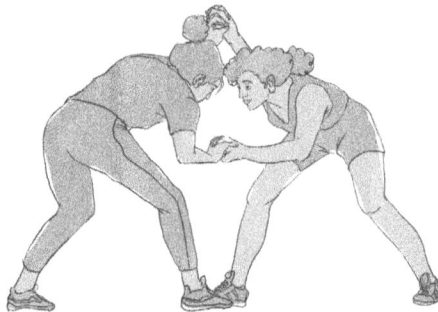

3) **Sit in the Sun with Face Covered.**
Sit in Easy Pose with a straight spine
and a light Neck Lock facing the sun.
Cover the face, except the forehead,
with the hands. Close the eyes and let
the sun shine on the forehead. Chant
HAR once per second. Use the tip
of the tongue to stimulate the upper
palate and pull the Navel Point with
each repetition. Continue for **13 ½
minutes**. (In the original class, the
recording "Tantric Har" by Simran
Kaur was played to keep the rhythm.)
TO END: Inhale deeply and
press the tip of the tongue firmly
against the upper palate. Suspend
the breath, exhale, and relax.

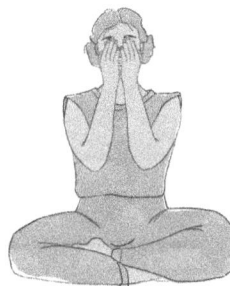

(36) Awaken the Chest and Nervous System

July 18, 1994

There are no pauses between exercises, unless indicated.

1) **Hit the Chest on 3.** Stand straight with the feet shoulder-width apart. Stretch the arms straight up, then out to the sides parallel to the ground, then hit the chest hard with both hands. Continue this 3 part movement at a pace of 3 seconds per cycle for **1 ½ minutes**.

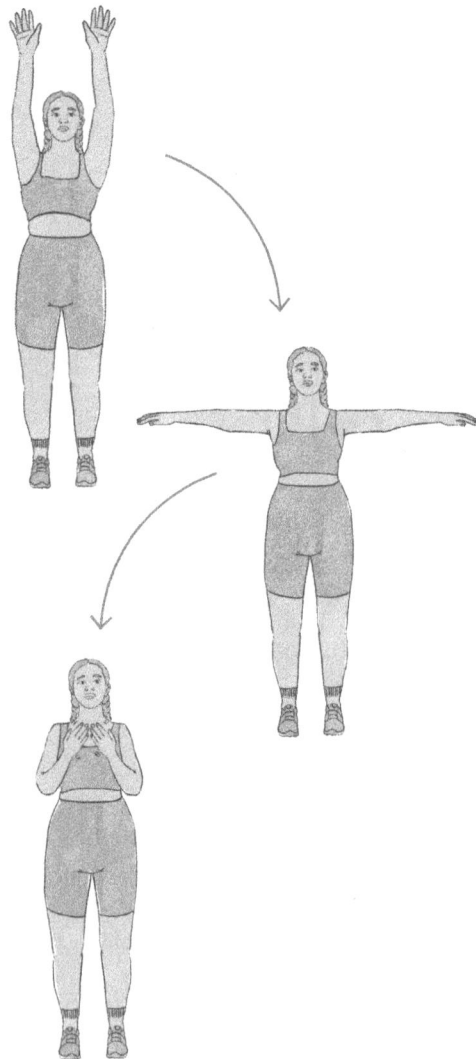

2) **Full Body Stretch.** Stand straight with the feet shoulder-width apart. Extend both arms straight up overhead, with palms forward and stretch your entire body up from your toes to your fingertips. Stretch higher, tighter, and farther with each count from 1 to 7, come onto your toes on 5, 6 and 7. Relax the stretch and bring the feet to ground and hands to the sides on the 8th count. Continue this cycle for **3 minutes**.

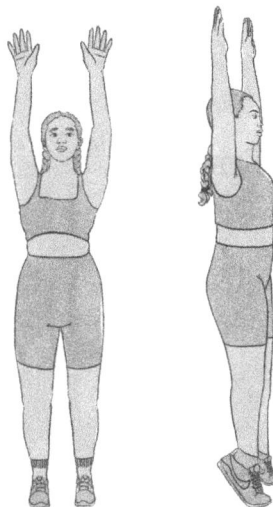

3) **Bhangra Dance.** Stand up and dance to the music. Make fists with both hands and alternately swing the arms across the body as you dance. Shift the weight from one foot to the other so that one foot is always off the ground. Open up the hips and move wildly for **6 ½ minutes.** (In the original class, Bhangra music was played.)

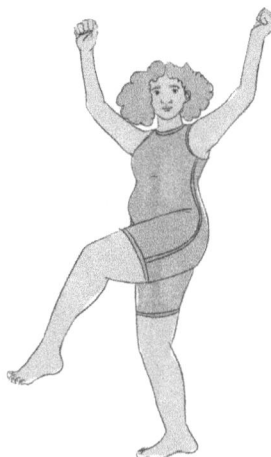

4) **Partner Wrestle.** ▲ Choose a partner, and begin to wrestle. Try to take the other person down, and pin them to the ground. Continue for **1 minute.**

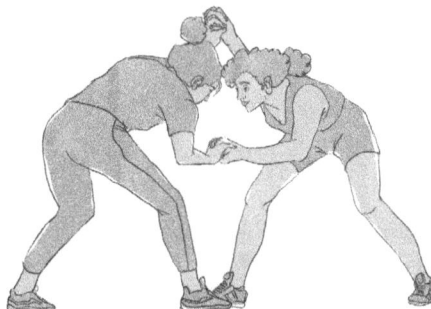

continue on next page »

5) Har Meditation with Clapping.
Sit in Easy Pose with a straight spine
and a light Neck Lock. Close the
eyes and chant **HAR.** Clap the hands
on each repetition and stimulate
the upper palate with the tip of the
tongue. Chant from the heart for
8 ½ minutes. (In the original class,
the recording "Tantric Har" by Simran
Kaur was played to keep the rhythm.)
TO END: Inhale deeply and relax.

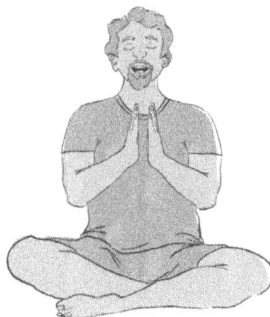

**6) Prayer Pose with Arms
Extended.** Remain in Easy Pose
and extend the arms straight up
with the hands in Prayer Pose. Sit
in stillness and meditate. Feel your
grace and capacity to endure. Keep
going and experience the power of
your endurance for **4 minutes**.

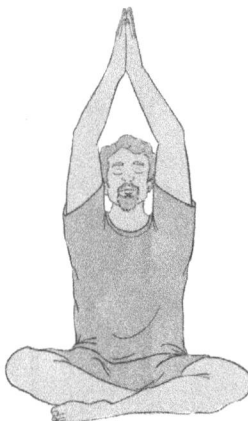

(37) Vibrant Vitality Series

July 19, 1994

There are no pauses between exercises.

1) **Standing Sat Kriya.** Stand straight with the feet hip-width apart. Interlock the hands overhead with the index fingers pointing up. Pull the arms upward and apply Neck Lock. Chant **SAT** as you squeeze the Navel Point in and up, chant **NAAM** as you release it. Move the navel with force (chant 8 times per 10 seconds) for **1 minute**. *This exercise works on the kidneys by moving the navel. Sat Kriya and the following exercise, are excellent to practice in bed before getting up.*

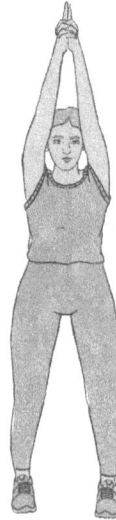

2) **Pelvic Movement Series.** a) Lie on the back with the arms by the sides. Keep the arms, legs, head and shoulders on the ground and raise the pelvis up and drop for **1 minute**. b) Remain on the back and move the entire spine from top to bottom in a rolling wave. Continue for **30 seconds**. c) Bounce the lower spine, legs and pelvis, up and down. Move quickly and powerfully for **30 seconds**. d) Bring the knees into the chest and wrap the arms around the knees. Lift the head up and bring the nose toward the knees. Rock back and forth on the spine from shoulder to hip for **30 seconds**.

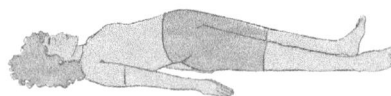

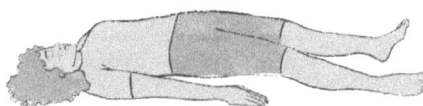

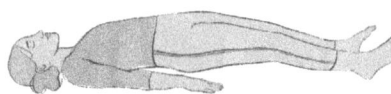

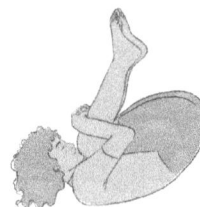

3) **Bhangra Dance.** Stand up and dance to the music. Make fists with both hands and alternately swing the arms across the body as you dance. Hop from one foot to the other so that only one foot touches the ground at a time. Continue for **4 minutes**. (In the original class, Bhangra music was played.)

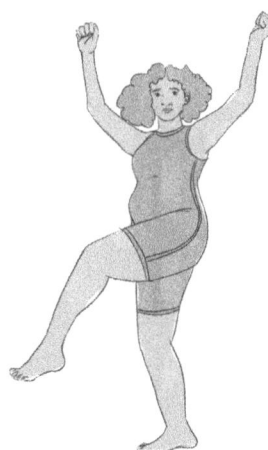

continue on next page »

4) **Sit in the Sun.** Sit in Easy Pose with a straight spine and a light Neck Lock facing the sun. Relax the elbows by the sides, bring the forearms up, and angle the palms toward the sun. Close the eyes and let the sun shine on the eyelids and forehead. Meditate for **7 minutes**[12].

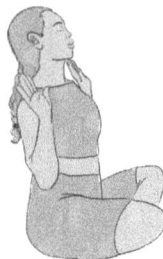

5) **Meditate and Move.** a) Place both hands on the Heart Center, one on top of the other. Close the eyes and meditate for **30 seconds**. b) Remain in the posture and meditatively move the body to the beat of the drum. Continue for **2 minutes**. (In the original class, Punjabi Drums were played to keep the rhythm.) *Relax the body and let it move naturally to the beat.*

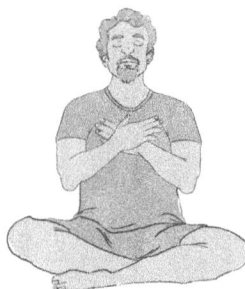

6) **Free Dance.** Keeping the eyes closed, stand up, and dance freely to uplifting music. Sing along and move as you feel. Continue for **6 minutes**. *If doing this exercise in a group setting, hold hands with a partner and dance together for the final 2 minutes.*

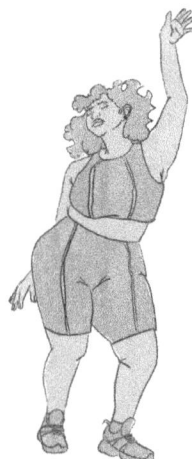

12 In the original class, an unavailable recording of "Siri Ram, Siri Ram, Siri Ram Haray" by an unknown artist was played.

7) Sit in the Sun with Face Covered.
Sit in a meditative posture facing
the sun. Cover the face with the
hands, leaving the forehead exposed.
Meditate for **6 ½ minutes**. Then
inhale deeply, exhale and relax.

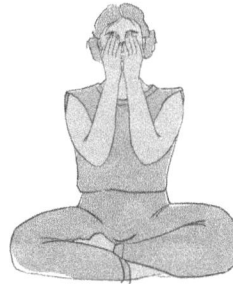

(38) Unveiling Inner Radiance and Balance

July 20, 1994

There are no pauses between exercises, unless indicated.

1) **Torso Circles.** Sit in Easy Pose, stretch the arms straight up, hands interlocked with the Jupiter (index) fingers extended. Move powerfully from the hips in large circles for **2 minutes**. *This exercise is very good for the spine.*

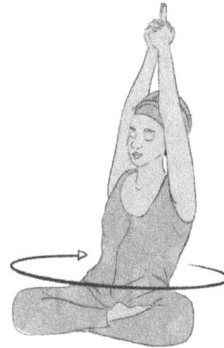

2) **Sufi Grind.** Remain in Easy Pose and place the hands on the knees. Lift the rib cage and, keeping the head, shoulders, rib cage as stable as possible, move the pelvis in circles. Isolate the movement to the pelvis. Move powerfully for **1 ½ minutes**.

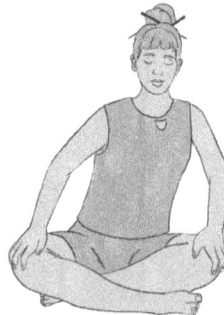

3) **Back Rolls.** Lie on the back and bring the knees to the chest, wrapping the arms around them. Rock back and forth on the spine from shoulder to hip for **1 ½ minutes**.

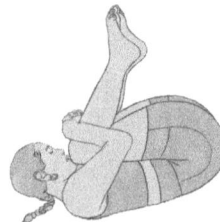

4) Har Meditation and Hit Chest.
Sit in Easy Pose with a straight spine,
a light Neck Lock and eyes closed.
Chant **HAR** and hit the Heart Center
with alternating hands, creating a
drum beat. Continue at a pace of one
hit per second for **11 ½ minutes**.
(In the original class, the recording
"Tantric Har" by Simran Kaur was
played to keep the rhythm.)
*This rhythm at the Heart Center helps
to release blocks from fear and anger.*

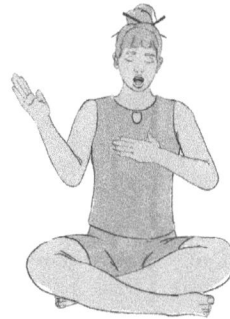

5) Ram Meditation. Remain in Easy
Pose with a straight spine and a light
Neck Lock. Relax the hands in the
lap. Become calm and concentrate
on the universe within. Meditate on
the Heart Chakra for **5 ½ minutes**.

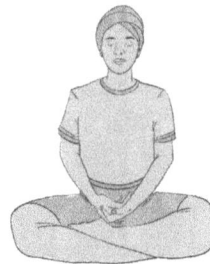

6) Free Dance. Stand up and dance
intuitively for **6 minutes**. Relax[13].
*If doing this exercise in a group setting,
hold hands and dance with a partner.*

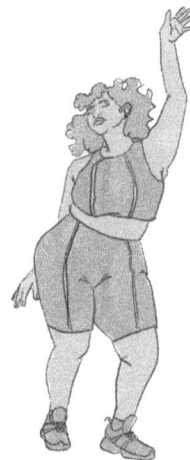

13 In the original class, an unavailable recording of "Siri
Ram, Siri Ram, Siri Ram Haray" by an unknown artist
was played.

(39) Tapping into Body Wisdom

July 22, 1994

There are no pauses between exercises.

1) **Hips Side-to-Side.** Stand straight with the feet hip-width apart. Fold forward and support your weight with the hands on the knees. Move the hips from side to side vigorously for **1 ½ minutes**.

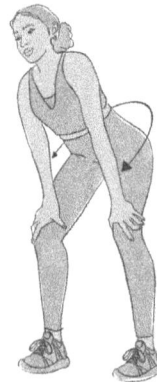

2) **Stand and Touch Ground.** Stand straight with the feet shoulder-width apart. Bend forward from the hips and hit the ground with both hands, then come up with the arms straight up overhead. Keep the legs straight and move powerfully for **8 minutes**.

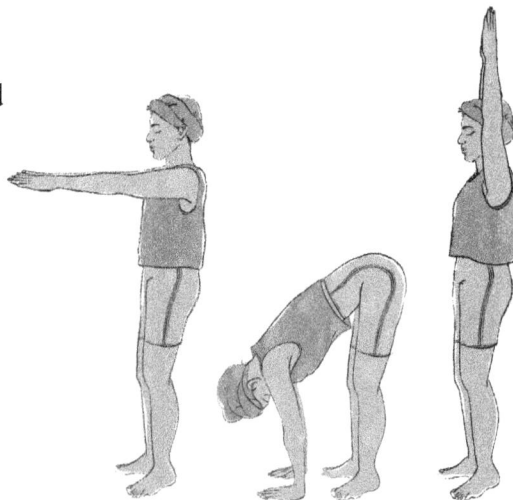

3) **Sit, Lay, Stand Series.** Sit in Easy Pose. Quickly lie down flat on the stomach. Then quickly stand up. Continue this three-part movement (1 cycle per 10 seconds) for **4 minutes**.

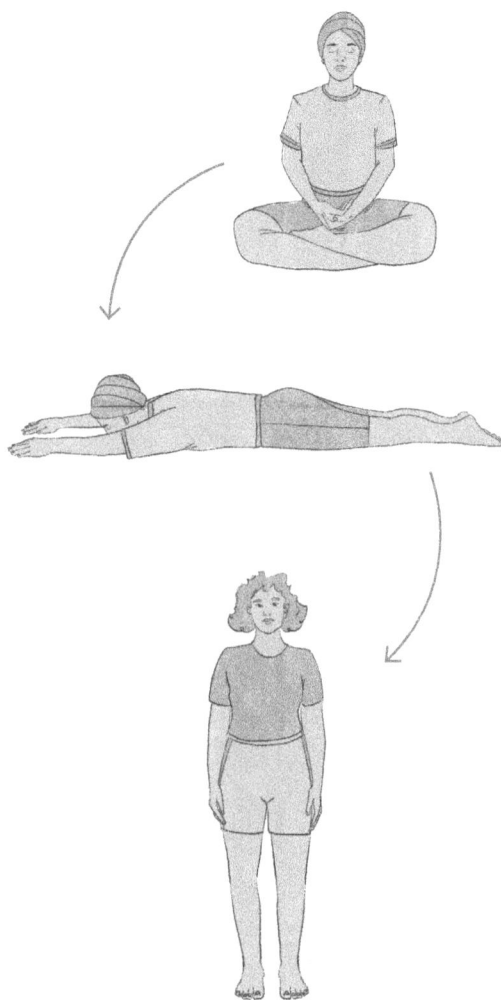

continue on next page »

4) **Bhangra Dance.** a) Stand up and dance to the music. Alternately move the hands from the hips to place fists on the rib cage as you hop from one foot to the other so that only one foot touches the ground at a time. Continue for **4 minutes**. b) Swing the arms back and forth alongside the body. Move the arms powerfully as you dance for **8 minutes**. (In the original class, Bhangra music was played.)
c) Chant **HAR** loudly as you dance. Continue for **14 minutes**. (In the original class, the recording "Tantric Har" by Simran Kaur was played.)

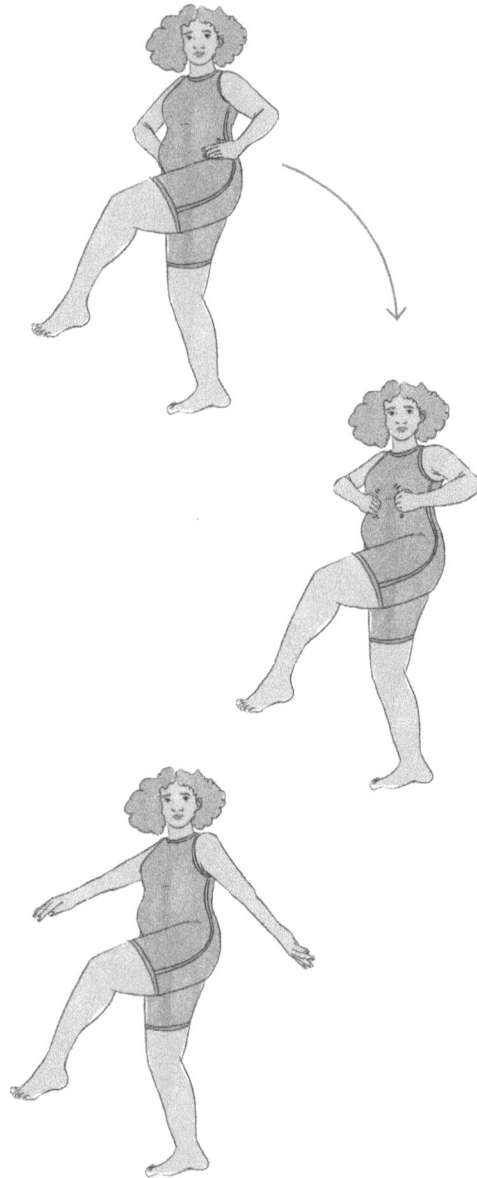

5) **Sit in the Sun.** Sit in Easy Pose with a straight spine and a light Neck Lock facing the sun. Relax the elbows by the sides, bring the forearms up, and angle the palms toward the sun. Close the eyes and let the sun shine on the eyelids and forehead. Meditate for **6 minutes**.

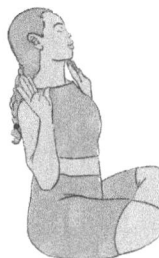

6) **Sphinx Pose.** Sit on the heels in Rock Pose. Bend forward and place the elbows and forearms on the ground. Lift the head and look up. Hold the posture for **1 minute**. *This posture fosters longevity.*

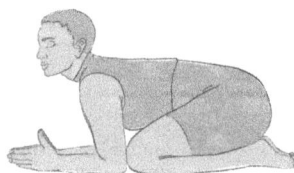

(40) Stimulating Circulation and Vitality

July 25, 1994

There are no pauses between exercises.

1) **Standing Torso Twists.** Stand straight with the feet shoulder-width apart. Stretch both arms out straight to the sides, parallel to the ground, palms facing down. Twist the body from left to right using the power and momentum of the arms. Keep the feet firmly planted on the ground, the arms stretched out from the shoulder, and move with force for **2 ½ minutes**.

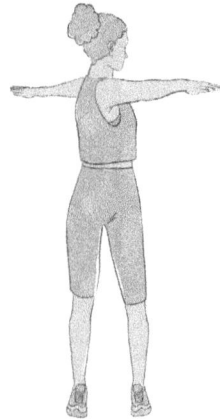

2) **Arm Circles.** Stand straight with the feet shoulder-width apart. Interlock the hands together in front of the body with the arms straight. Make very large circles with the arms and allow the whole body to move with them. Keep the arms straight and move fast and powerfully for **2 ½ minutes**.

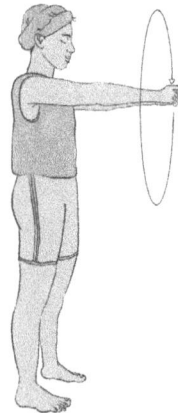

3) **Chop Wood.** Stand straight with the feet shoulder-width apart and the hands interlocked overhead. Keeping the arms in line with the spine, bend forward from the hips, bringing the arms between the legs, then come back up and lean backward. Continue to alternate between the two positions for **2 minutes**.

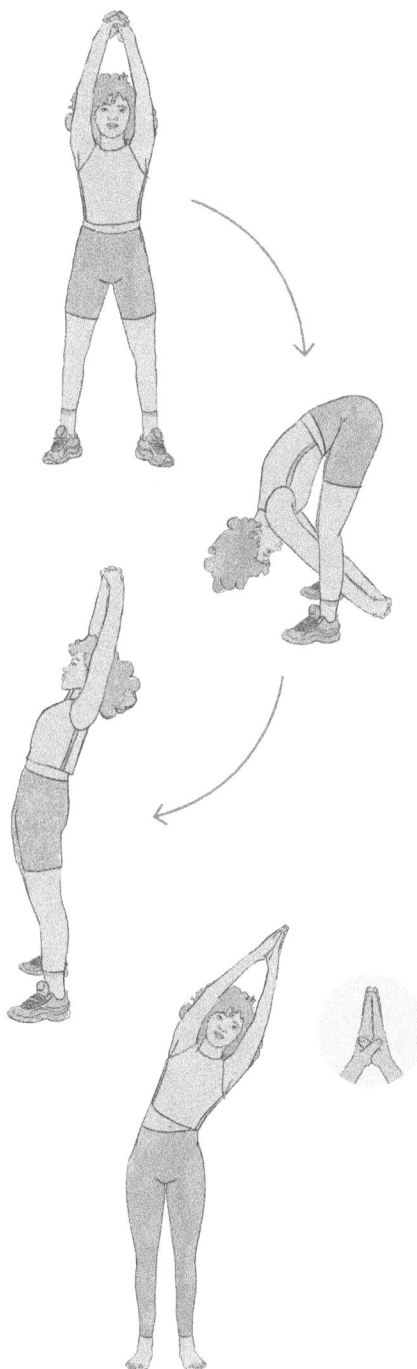

4) **Standing Side Bends.** Stand straight with the feet shoulder-width apart. Bring the palms together overhead and cross the thumbs. Bend sideways from left to right for **5 minutes**.

continue on next page »

5) **Run and Chant.** Run laps around your space and chant **HAR** as you run. Continue for **14 ½ minutes**. (In the original class, the recording "Tantric Har" by Simran Kaur was played.) *If practicing outside, run laps around your space. Chanting loudly as you run releases anger and increases pranic energy.*

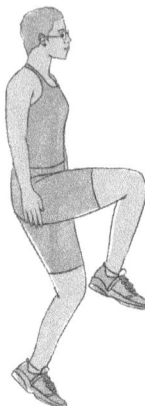

6) **Sit in the Sun.** Sit in Easy Pose with a straight spine and a light Neck Lock facing the sun. Relax the elbows by the sides, bring the forearms up, and angle the palms toward the sun. Close the eyes and let the sun shine on the eyelids and forehead. Sing for **6 minutes**.

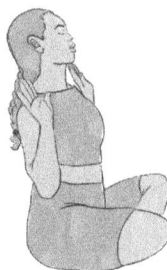

7) **Tube of Light Meditation.** Remain in the posture. Hypnotize yourself and imagine the spine to be a shining, fluorescent tube of light and the head a bright light bulb. Meditatively illuminate these two parts of the body for **17 minutes**. (In the original class, the recording "Meditation" by Wahe Guru Kaur was played.) TO END: Inhale deeply, stretch the arms up, and tighten every muscle of the body; hold for **10-15 seconds**. Exhale. Repeat this breath **3 times total**. Shake the arms and hands out, then relax.

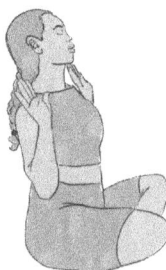

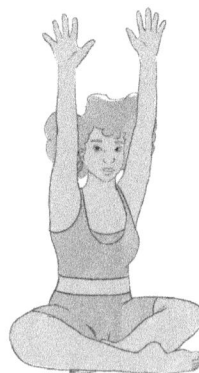

(41) Energizing Jumping Sequence

July 26, 1994

There are no pauses between exercises, unless indicated.

1) **Jumping Jacks.** Stand straight with the arms at your sides. Jump and open the legs wide as you bring both arms straight up and clap the hands over the head (1 clap per second). Jump again and bring the feet together and the arms down to your sides. Continue alternately jumping from one position to the other in a continuous motion for **3 minutes**.

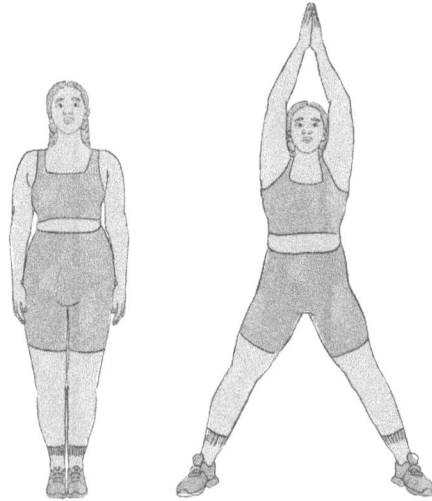

2) **Jump on All Fours.** Stand on your hands and feet with equal weight. Jump up and down so all four leave and return to the ground at the same time. Continue for **1 minute**.

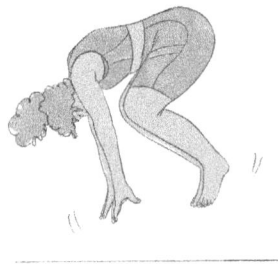

3) **Hop Kicks.** a) Stand with the feet shoulder-width apart and the hands on the hips. Hop onto one leg while kicking the other leg forward and up. Continue alternately kicking the legs for **1 minute.** b) Swing the arms back and forth in rhythm with the movement for **3 minutes**. (In the original class, the recording "Tantric Har" by Simran Kaur was played to keep the rhythm.)

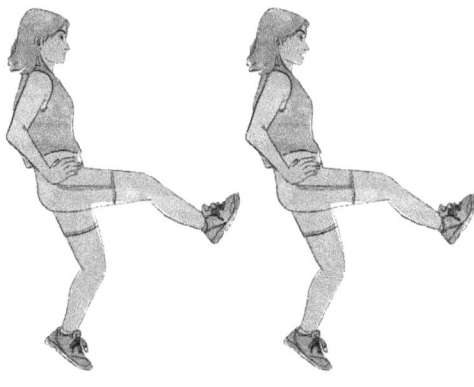

4) **Running.** Run laps around your space for **12 ½ minutes**. (In the original class, the recording "Tantric Har" by Simran Kaur was played to keep the rhythm.)
If practicing inside, run in place.

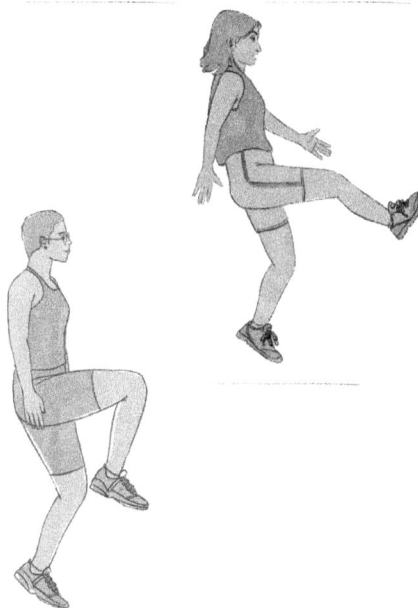

5) **Sit in the Sun.** Sit in Easy Pose with a straight spine and a light Neck Lock facing the sun. Relax the elbows by the sides, bring the forearms up, and angle the palms toward the sun. Close the eyes and let the sun shine on the eyelids and forehead. Meditate for **4 minutes**. TO END: Inhale deeply and exhale **3 times**. Relax.

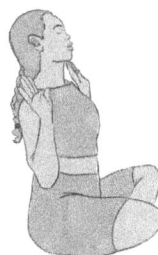

(42) Energize Body and Spirit

July 28, 1994

There are no pauses between exercises.

1) **Running.** Run laps around your space. Continue for **12 minutes**. (In the original class, Punjabi Drums were played to keep the rhythm.)

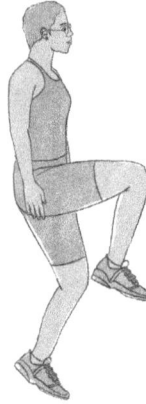

2) **Rope Pulls.** Sit in Easy Pose. Alternately reach forward as if grasping a rope, then make a fist and pull back towards the body. Draw the fists in powerfully for **3 ½ minutes**. *Moving powerfully in this exercise opens up the rib cage.*

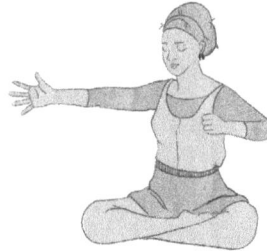

3) **Bhangra Dance.** Stand up and dance to the music. Keep the arms raised above the Heart Center, move the shoulders up and down and shift the weight from one foot to the other so that one foot is always off the ground. Continue for **6 minutes**. (In the original class, Bhangra music was played.)

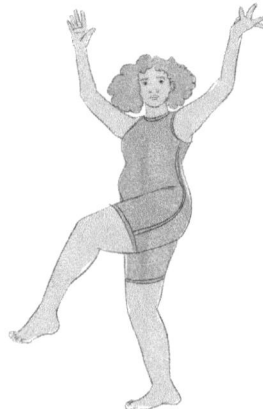

4) **Jumping Jacks.** Stand straight with the arms at your sides. Jump and open the legs wide as you bring both arms straight up and clap the hands over the head (1 clap per second). Jump again and bring the feet together and the arms down to your sides. Continue alternately jumping from one position to the other in a continuous motion for **3 minutes**. (In the original class, Bhangra music was played.) *This exercise is very good for the nervous system.*

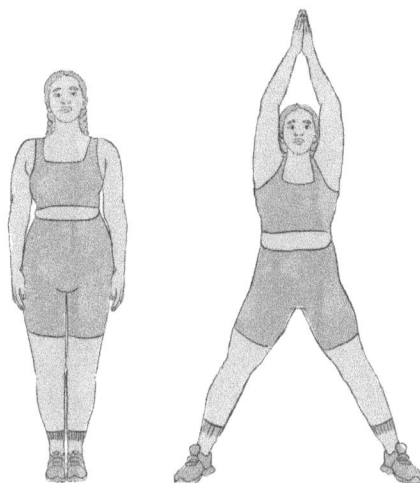

5) **Sit in the Sun.** Sit in Easy Pose with a straight spine and a light Neck Lock facing the sun. Relax the elbows by the sides, bring the forearms up, and angle the palms toward the sun. Close the eyes and let the sun shine on the eyelids and forehead. Meditate for **31 minutes**. (In the original class, the recordings "Ghor Dukhyung" by Guru Raj Kaur, "Jai Te Gung" by an unknown artist, "Raakhe Rakhanhaar" by Singh Kaur, and "Deh Shiva Bar Mohe" by Anuradha Paudwal were played.)

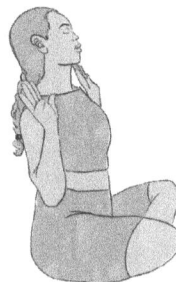

(43) Seven Steps for Health

July 29, 1994

There are no pauses between exercises.

1) **Parallel Forward Bend.** Stand straight with the feet shoulder-width apart. Place the hands on the hips. Bend forward so the upper body is parallel to the ground. The head is up, not in Neck Lock. Stretch forward with the arms and head and back with the hips; create a balance, keeping the legs and spine straight for **1 ½ minutes**.

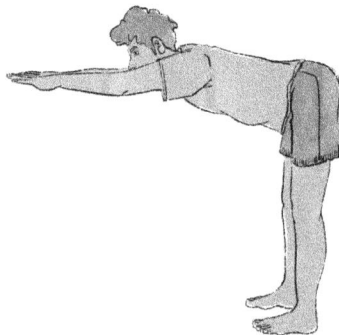

2) **Hammer Circle.** Stand straight with the feet slightly wider than the hips. Bend forward from the hips so the upper body is parallel to the ground and let both arms hang loosely. Swing the arms in circles with the body; to the right, around and back down. Stop at the starting point, change directions, and circle to the left. Alternate directions for **1 minute**.

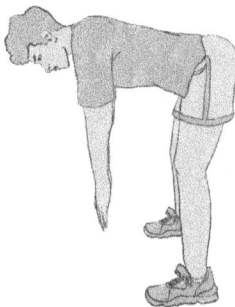

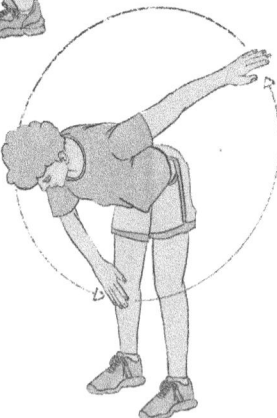

222

3) **Jump on All Fours.** Stand on your hands and feet with equal weight. Jump up and down so all four leave and return to the ground at the same time. Continue for **1 minute.**

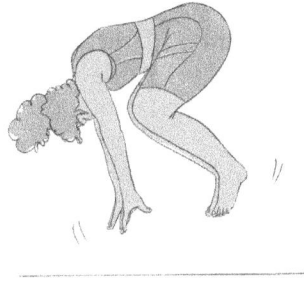

4) **Pelvic Tilt.** Stand up straight with the feet shoulder-width apart. Raise both arms straight overhead with the palms facing forward. Lean the upper body forward and backward 40 degrees from the hips, keeping the arms aligned. Tilt the pelvis back as you lean forward and forward as you lean back. Continue for **1 minute**.

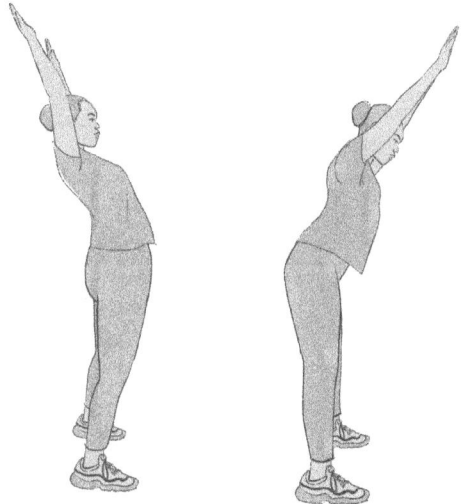

5) **Leap Run.** Run laps around your space. Jump slightly with each step and use long strides for **2 ½ minutes**.

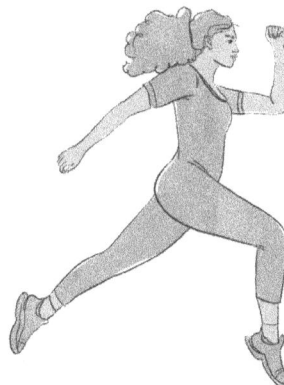

continue on next page »

6) **Har Meditation.** Sit in Easy
Pose with a straight spine and a light
Neck Lock. Bring the hands beside
the shoulders, palms facing forward.
Open up the rib cage by pushing the
chest out. Focus the eyes at the tip
of the nose. Chant **HAR** in rhythm
for **5 ½ minutes**. (In the original
class, the recording "Tantric Har"
by Simran Kaur was played.)

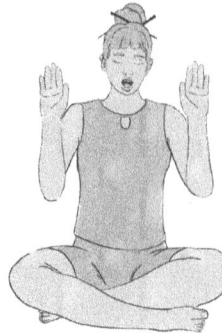

7) **Stretching Series.** Lie on the back in Corpse Pose. a) Stretch the arms out to the sides from the shoulders. Bring one knee into the chest and, keeping the arms and shoulders on the ground, roll it over to the opposite side for a Cat Stretch. Switch sides and continue for **30 seconds**. b) Stand on the hands and knees and flex the spine up and down in Cat/Cow for **30 seconds**. c) Lie on the stomach with the arms stretched forward on the ground. Totally relax and sleep for **1 minute**. d) Roll onto the side and come up standing. Bend forward and touch the toes briefly, then come up standing with the hands in Prayer Pose. Say a silent prayer for **1 ½ minutes**.

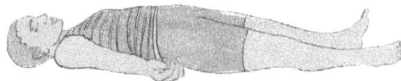

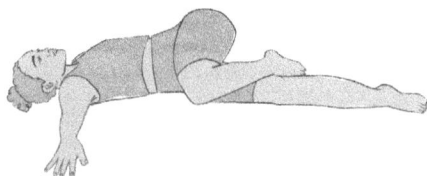

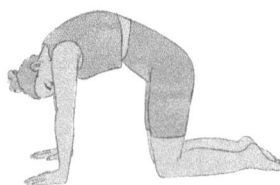

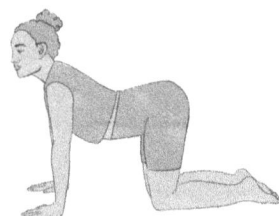

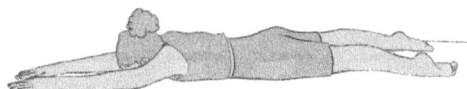

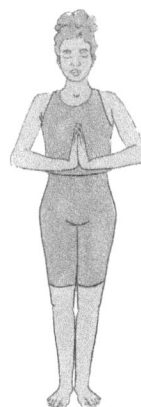

APPENDIX

AQUARIAN SADHANA MANTRAS

The following sequence of mantras was given in 1992 with instructions to use them for early morning Aquarian Sadhana until the beginning of the Aquarian Age. After that time, we could keep that particular Sadhana, or develop a new one. After the beginning of the Aquarian Age (after November 2011), this was discussed among Teacher Trainers, and it was decided to keep this sadhana as it is so it could be practiced in group consciousness by everyone around the world.

1. The Adi Shakti Mantra (7 minutes)

Ek Ong Kaar Sat Naam Siri Wha-hay Guroo
One Creator created this Creation. Truth is His Name. Great beyond description is the Divine Intelligence of Infinite Wisdom.

The cornerstone of morning sadhana is an Ashtang Mantra, the Adi Shakti Mantra, also called Long Ek Ong Kars or Morning Call. This mantra initiates the kundalini, initiating the relationship between our soul and the Universal Soul. Long Ek Ong Kaars are chanted without musical accompaniment, whereas the six mantras that follow may be chanted using various melodies with or without instrumental accompaniment.

2. Waah Yantee, Kar Yantee (7 minutes)

Waah Yantee Kaar Yantee,
Jagadootpatee,
Aadak It Whaa-Haa,
Brahmaaday Trayshaa Guroo
It Whaa-Hay Guroo

Great Macroself, Creative Self. All that is creative through time. All that is the Great One. Three aspects of God: Brahma, Vishnu, Mahesh (Shiva). That is Wahe Guru.

This mantra uses the words of Patanjali. It represents thousands of years of prayer. Through it, we call directly on the macroself, beyond the gunas, beyond creation.

3. The Mul Mantra (7 minutes)

Ek Ong Kaar
Sat Naam
Kartaa Purkh
Nirbho Nirvair
Akaal Moorat
Ajoonee
Saibung
Gur Prasaad
Jap!
Aad Such
Jugaad Such
Hai Bhee Such
Nanak Hosee Bhee Such

One Creator, Creation
I identify with Truth Doer of Everything
Fearless, revengeless
Undying, unborn
Self-illumined, Self existent
Guru's grace (gift)
REPEAT (Chant)
True in the beginning
True through all time
True even now
Nanak says Truth shall ever be

The Mul (Root) Mantra gives an experience of the depth and consciousness of the soul. This mantra expands creativity and projects us into action in line with the Creator, and our destiny. In chanting the Mul Mantra, (a) leave a slight space (not a breath) between ajoonee and saibhang. Do not run the words together; and (b) emphasize the "ch" sound at the end of the word "such." This adds power.

4. Sat Siree, Siree Akal (7 minutes)

**Sat Siree Siree Akaal
Siree Akaal Mahaa Akaal
Mahaa Akaal Sat Naam
Akaal Moorat Wha-Hay Guroo**

Great Truth, Respected Undying
Respected Undying, Great Deathless
Great Deathless, Truth Identified (Named)
Deathless Image of God, Great beyond description is Divine Wisdom

This is the Mantra for the Aquarian Age. We vibrate at the frequency of this Age. Through it, we declare that we are timeless, deathless beings.

5. Rakhe Rakhan Har (7 minutes)

**Rakhay Rakhanhaar Aap Ubaariun
Gur Kee Pairee Paa-eh Kaaj Savaariun
Hoaa Aap Dayaal Manho Na Visaariun
Saadh Janaa Kai Sung Bhavjal Taariun
Saakat Nindak Dusht Khin Maa-eh Bidaariun
Tis Saahib Kee Tayk Naanak Manai Maa-Eh
Jis Simrat Sukh Ho-Eh Saglay Dookh Jaa-Eh**

You, Yourself are caring for us all and taking us across, Uplifting and giving us excellence. You gave us the touch of the lotus feet of the Guru, and all our affairs are covered. You are merciful, kind, compassionate; and our minds never forget

You. In the company of conscious people, you take us from misfortune. You remove any enemies from our path. You are my anchor. Nanak, keep firm in your mind, by meditating and repeating His Name I feel peaceful and happy and all my pain departs.

This is a shabd of protection against all negative forces which move against one's walk on the path of destiny, both inner and outer. It cuts like a sword through every opposing vibration, thought, word, and action. It is part of the evening prayer of the Sikhs (Rehiras). Rakhe Rakhan Har was composed by Guru Arjan, the Fifth Guru.

6. Wahe Guru Wahe Jio (22 minutes)

Wha-Hay Guroo, Wha-Hay Guroo, Wha-Hay Guroo, Wha-Hay Jeeo

Chant this mantra sitting in Vir Asan: sitting on the left heel with the right knee up, right foot flat on the ground and hands in Prayer Pose. Eyes are open, focused at the Tip of the Nose. This begins to take away fear. Deeply listen to your own chanting. Wahe Guru is a mantra of ecstasy. Loosely translated, we could say, "Wow, God is great!" or "indescribably great is the Infinite, Ultimate Intelligence." Jeeo is an affectionate but still respectful variation of the word Jee which means soul. We establish ourselves for victory and the right to excel.

7. Guru Ram Das Chant (5 minutes)

Guroo Guroo Wha-Hay Guroo Guroo Raam Das Guroo

In praise of the consciousness of Guru Ram Das, invoking that spiritual light, guidance, and protective grace. We are filled with humility, and emotional relaxation.

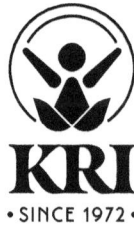

A Kundalini Yoga Global Community
KUNDALINIRESEARCHINSTITUTE.ORG